Dr Gerry Bennett trained at the Welsh National School of Medicine and is a Fellow of the Royal College of Physicians. He was Vice-Chairman of Age Concern Greater London from 1991 to 1993. He is Reader at the Royal London Medical College, Visiting Professor Healthcare of the Elderly Queen's University Belfast and Medical Director Tower Hamlets Healthcare NHS Trust. He has published widely and his writing and special research interests include chronic wounds and elder abuse. He is the Chair of the charity Action on Elder Abuse.

J. Marshall.

GW00368190

Alzheimer's Disease

AND OTHER

Dementias

Dr Gerry Bennet

Illustrated by
Jennie Smith

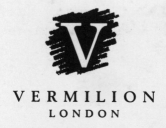

VERMILION
LONDON

First published by Macdonald Optima in 1994

Reprinted 1994

1 3 5 7 9 10 8 6 4 2

This edition published in the United Kingdom in 1996 by Vermilion
an imprint of Ebury Press

Random House UK Ltd
Random House
20 Vauxhall Bridge Road
London SW1V 2SA

Random House Australia (Pty) Ltd
20 Alfred Street, Milsons Point, Sydney,
New South Wales 2061, Australia

Random House New Zealand Limited
18 Poland Road, Glenfield,
Auckland 10, New Zealand

Random House, South Africa (Pty) Limited
Box 2263, Rosebank 2121, South Africa

Random House UK Limited Reg. No. 954009

A CIP catalogue record for this book is available from the British
Library.

ISBN 0 09 181280 1

Printed and bound in Great Britain by Mackays of Chatham, plc

Papers used by Vermilion are natural, recyclable products made
from wood grown in sustainable forests.

Contents

Acknowledgements

There are four people who in their different ways contributed to the writing of this book: my parents Madeleine and Jim Bennett who sacrificed all when I was young and who were always there when I needed them; Hywel, my companion; and Professor Peter Millard, a truly worthy medical mentor.

I would also like to thank Hilary, Brenda and Jackie for their help with the original manuscript and Jo for her help with this edition as well as Carrie and Richard Moyes for their past help.

Finally I would like to mention Dr Isabel Moyes who sadly died whilst I was writing the first edition and whose help and enthusiasm was much appreciated.

*This book is dedicated to
Eric Neils who died in June 1988*

Preface

Our society is growing older, with 17 per cent of people aged over 65. This fact should be seen as a major social and medical achievement, brought about by improved standards in housing, sewerage control, nutrition, education, and general medical care within the last two centuries. Yet old age or being older is rarely viewed as a success story; indeed many people fear growing old. Why do we tend to have such a negative view of a period of time which for many of us will amount to a third of our entire lifespan? In part the reasons lie within our perception of the elderly and especially the media portrayal of older people. Stories about fit elderly people living fulfilling independent lives are not the stuff of headlines and do not sell copy. Instead the reports are of muggings, a health service failing the needs of the sick and old, and the awful consequences of poverty, poor housing and isolation.

Obviously, a contented old age is somewhat dependent upon adequate finances (usually solely the State pension), good housing and social contact; the achievement of these conditions for all elderly people must therefore be stridently pursued. Simply reporting what is bad in our society is counterproductive: it leads to a biased and misleading view about what being older really means for the majority of elderly people. It perpetuates myths, especially about the ageing process, which can have dire medical and social consequences, for example confusion = dementia = senility, and that old people should expect to be incontinent, fall down and have poor sight and hearing.

Ageism (a detrimental view of old age) is widespread. In our society retirement means loss. There is the loss of status, and the label 'pensioner' or 'senior citizen' which is usually accompanied by a significant loss of income. Advertising (holidays, cars, clothes and other consumer goods – apart from vitamin pills and laxatives) is seldom aimed at the older person; only the young and middle-aged are seen as having any spending power and hence worth. When it comes to health care the elderly are seen as distinctly second-class citizens. Private health care schemes are not interested in attracting clients over the age of 65 and are quite open in stating that the National Health Service is the place for the elderly and those with any 'chronic' disorders. Many hospitals still house their elderly patients in old workhouse sections, albeit a bit tarted up, and they are usually the last group to move out of these surroundings into any new developments. Care of the chronically sick elderly, where the specialty of Geriatric Medicine was born, is now no longer seen by the government as part of NHS care at all, with parts of the country having no specialised continuing care for the elderly. This type of care is being privatised wholesale.

Professionals in the health service and lay people alike use the term geriatric almost as a term of abuse – when did you last hear of a child being called a paediatric? The term geriatric refers to a branch of medicine that deals with the problems of old age, hence the Department of Geriatric Medicine, etc. Geriatricians are specialists in this field of medicine, but because the word geriatric has been so abused most health care workers are abandoning it and using terms such as 'health care of the elderly', 'medicine of old age' and so on. This emphasis on words is important because it is another aspect of ageism. The medical problems of older people have only comparatively recently attracted the interest of doctors, nurses and other health workers. General practitioners have lagged behind in gaining this new knowledge and there is a sad lack of informative and enlightened articles in the lay press. It is not surprising then that the modern concepts of what is normal ageing and what is ill health have not reached the client.

Elderly people themselves, their relatives and carers still have appallingly low expectations of their health prospects and even a lower awareness of their health rights. Falling over, becoming incontinent and having trouble walking are accepted without question as being part of growing old. Becoming confused or 'senile' or 'demented' is seen as the worst but also an unavoidable aspect of old age. If this book does nothing else but get the message across to as many people as possible that falls, incontinence, immobility and especially confusion, are symptoms of illness and not age then it will have been a success.

There are thousands of elderly people suffering the pain and indignity of these conditions, merely accepting them. There are still doctors and other professionals who when confronted with these symptoms will tell the patient, 'what do you expect? It's just your age and nothing can be done'. This is, to put it politely, nonsense, and the professional should be told so. Obviously not every condition can be cured, but that fact can only be certain after all the treatable causes have been ruled out. It's time for 'grey power' when it comes to demanding that the health problems of the elderly are recognised and tackled.

The following chapters deal in depth with the condition of confusion in elderly people. The size of the problem is outlined and the treatable and non-treatable causes are explained. The best way to get the health service and social services to help the client is outlined and there is a review of how new discoveries hold out hope for the future. Coping with an irreversibly confused person can be a daunting task and this aspect is looked at from the carer's point of view with the emphasis on the practical help available and how to get it. A happy and contented old age is a success story and must be seen as such; demystifying some of its health problems is one way forward.

1

The rising tide

If figures and statistics were the proof of success then old age would be a surefire winner. Less than a hundred years ago only 4 per cent of the population were aged 65 or over. This figure is now about 17 per cent or roughly 8 million elderly people. How has this explosion in numbers come about? It is the result of a set of complex and intermingled factors. Our basic living conditions have greatly improved and the majority of us take for granted piped water, flushing toilets, homes with lighting and heating, as well as fairly unlimited basic food provision. This improvement in our social situation has meant that our general health has also improved and we no longer suffer the ravages of epidemics such as cholera and bubonic plague, which were commonplace in grossly insanitary conditions.

Advances in medicine have played a less dramatic role. Nonetheless they have helped in bringing down the previously horrendous infant mortality figures. Families used to have huge numbers of children, partly to try and ensure that a few made it through the deadly pitfalls of infancy. Most babies born now can confidently be expected to live to at least 75 years of age. A sophisticated health service has also ensured that people do not die of common conditions such as appendicitis or complicated fractured bones, as used to be the case. We now take for granted antibiotics, operations and even spare-part surgery. Trends are for families to have fewer children, but virtually all of them will live to be old and many to be very old indeed. Obviously the total numbers of old people in a population will depend on the birth rate many years previously and any special factors that may have intervened.

In the UK we have reached the peak in total numbers of people over the age of 65 and indeed the numbers may drop slightly into the next century. However, within that total number is a group who are going to live to a very old age and this group is getting larger – the so-called old old. These people were born before the First World War and have reaped the benefits of the social and medical changes that have increased their life expectancy. However, the First World War will also be remembered for removing a generation of young men, leaving a large number of women to remain unmarried or widowed, and hence to enter old age much more isolated. This cohort of elderly destined to become very old will continue to rise towards the end of the century. This is not just an interesting demographic change but a profound challenge for our society.

The challenge is that this group of elderly people will make enormous demands on our health and social services. They will see their general practitioner more frequently and use more of the primary care teams services such as district nurse and, where available, chiropodist, etc. When admission is necessary they will spend longer in hospital and need complex multi-disciplinary assessment. In the community (where the vast numbers of old people always are) they will need increased amounts of support from specialist housing, social services and the voluntary sector. The needs of their carers will also have to be met. Although a small

UK population by age, 1981–2025 (in millions)

	all ages	over 75
1981	56.4	3.3
1987	56.9	3.8
1991	57.5	4.0
1996	58.3	4.2
2001	59.0	4.4
2006	59.3	4.4
2011	59.4	4.4
2025	60.0	5.3

percentage of the total numbers of old people, this group will need a disproportionate share of the resources if their needs are to be adequately covered.

If meeting the needs of a large number of very old people is a challenge, then meeting the needs of those within that group suffering from chronic confusion will be difficult indeed. Taken at face value the numbers involved seem enormous and overwhelming; even a multidisciplinary advisory group not used to overstatement called the impending challenge 'the rising tide'. The facts as they are currently known estimate that when the numbers of very old are at their peak there will be about one million old people with some form of dementia. This represents about one in ten of the total number of over 65s and one in five of the very old, i.e. 85+. The most recent research work done in this field suggests that these figures may be an overestimate, but even if correct the reverse is also true, that nine out of ten people over the age of 65 and four out of five of those aged over 85 will have no dementia at all.

Regardless of the final statistics, the numbers involved will still cause us formidable problems unless measures are taken now. Society as a whole and the health and social services in particular are not coping with the current numbers of old people, especially those who need specialist services such as those with dementia. Until the mid 1980s it was known that only 6 per cent of elderly people lived in any form of institution such as an old people's home or hospital long-stay ward. It was one of the lowest figures for institutional care in the developed world. The need for more care, in some form, was obviously not being met however, and when the government decided to pay for residential or nursing home care without compulsory assessment the flood gates opened. It is now estimated that 6 per cent of elderly people over 65 are now in institutional care, the huge increase being within the private sector. The cost to the government has been has been literally billions of pounds and precipitated the Care in the Community legislation (see chapter 8).

The remainder of elderly people live at home, many helped by their families, but at least ⅓ live alone. The UK has been looked upon as a world leader in its range of provision for elderly people, but as one who works in the system I see that the provision is breaking down and basic services that ensure a minimum quality of life and keep an individual at home with some form of independence are failing to be delivered. There are insufficient services for the elderly mentally frail and their carers now, few having access to day and night sitting services or respite care. Our institutions, when they can be used, are usually under-staffed and under-resourced. Carers, be they family or otherwise, keep our system from collapsing about our ears; they are the group that will face the biggest burdens when this 'rising tide' peaks. We fail them as we fail the sufferer – at our peril.

It is very easy to become insular when thinking about the age changes occurring in our society. We tend to see it from the perspective of an already advanced society used to the ideas of retirement, pensions and free or direct access to health and social care. Our debates are over the direction social policy should take, and the questions of whether the funding should be from the public or private sector. We should take some time, however to look at the more global aspects of this age change for it is not restricted to the so-called developed world. Though it may be slower in some areas than others, all the developing nations are also experiencing a fall in infant mortality and a rise in life expectancy. Many now have populations where the overwhelming number of people are children, destined to live to be old in countries where old people were a rarity. In 1900 approximately 1% of the world's population was aged over 65. Some countries such as China will have more older people than the entire current United States population and India will have an even greater percentage older population. Many nations are facing up to this prospect already and are developing schemes to cope with the numbers involved. India, Kenya and many Latin American countries are a few where highly organised programmes are already underway. They face enormous difficulties, often financial – these countries have to cope with huge national and international debts with no prospect of there being sufficient money available to finance pensions. Without some form of pension most people could not consider retiring.

The concept of retirement does not exist in developing countries for without work a person starves. As these countries become more industrialised they will undergo the same changes that we went through many years ago, with the younger members moving to the cities to find work, splitting the family networks and leaving the elderly isolated. In much of the developing world the concept of an institution for the old does not exist and culturally it is one that they do not want to introduce. Many such countries see themselves as being in the fortunate position of learning by our mistakes and it is true to say that they are spending what limited resources they have on keeping the elderly in the community and where possible using their accumulated skills and knowledge to help that community.

The fact that our life expectancy is rising has already been commented upon. It is now not that rare for someone to live to be 100 but it is still far from the norm. Some scientists believe that we are approaching the limit of life expectancy for most of us and that the few who surpass it by many years are in fact 'biologically elite'. They feel that our genetic make-up is programmed to self-destruct and that social and health trends have reached the limit to delay this. Many others feel that there is still great capacity for prolonging the overall life-span and point to research work on rats and mice that can considerably extend their life expectancy. The study of ageing – gerontology – is now a rapidly expanding field of scientific research. It has finally shed its image of quacks searching for the elixir of youth and is beginning to show that the ageing process is far more complicated than previously thought.

The old concept of wear and tear no longer holds true. Whatever the outcome – and I tend to feel that we have not seen the end of the rising life expectancy curve – we must ensure that the quality of life rather than the quantity remains the overriding principle. 'Add life to years'.

2

Acute confusion

Acute confusion in the elderly is a very common condition. 'Acute' can mean anything from something lasting only a few minutes to a state lasting up to three months. The point that must be stressed again and again, however, is that confusion is not dementia and that acute confusion in an old person is simply that person's way of presenting with an illness. The vast majority of acute confusional states in old people are fully reversible.

What do we mean by acute confusion? One of the best descriptive words for it is 'delirium'. One can then picture the sufferer being disorientated in time and place: they are not sure where they are and what time of day it is. Their mood is up and down, one minute calm and happy to cooperate and the next agitated and wanting to do inappropriate things. This is often called labile mood. The person's memory is usually poor and they can be quite drowsy at times. One of the most distressing features is the tendency to hallucinations and delusions. Hallucinations occur more easily if the person has poor eyesight and hearing, but they also tend to happen when the light is poor (the twilight times of dawn and evening). The condition of confusion occurring at twilight has been termed sundowner syndrome. Common objects get mistaken for something more sinister – the pattern on the carpet becomes a mass of crawling insects. Delusions are wrong ideas that the deluded person will not accept as wrong; you can talk and explain until you are blue in the face but the sufferer will still insist that they are right. Delusions can take many forms but in acute confusion they are usually shortlived. They may be slightly comical in that the sufferer insists that a number 48 bus is due in their bedroom any minute to take them to the shops. Sometimes they are more distressing, especially when the person insists, for example, that their food is poisoned or that one of their carers is going to harm them. These are known as paranoid delusions, paranoia being a mental state where you wrongly think that you are going to be harmed.

People with acute confusional states are not usually aggressive. Occasionally violence in the form of hitting out occurs, usually as the result of the confused person being restrained from doing something which is going to be harmful to them. If agitated, the person's speech is often affected; sentences don't get finished as they rush onto something else, or the drowsiness can make the speech a little slurred. Conditions that cause confusional states to come on very suddenly (such as infections) often cause the person to look and feel unwell. They may be flushed and warm to the touch, even sweating. They may complain of very vague aches and pains as well as having no appetite. Nausea and vomiting can occur and the confusion may be accompanied by weakness and lethargy. Sometimes no other symptoms occur and yet an underlying illness is still present.

You will realise from what I have described above that the condition can be very frightening for the carers. Suddenly they may be dealing with a relative who not only appears unwell but is difficult to handle. The confusion may also be accompanied by the other symptoms (weakness, etc.) or by incontinence. The carer may be accused of nasty deeds, or have a difficult job stopping their relative trying to leave the house or doing other inappropriate acts. Sometimes there is nothing as florid as the above descriptions, just a feeling from the carers that all is not right and that the person, in some hard to define way, is not their usual self. This usually stems from some odd behaviour or speech, which indicates that the person is confused.

Causes of acute confusion

The following list shows some of the more common causes of acute confusion in elderly people. The main ones are discussed in more detail explaining the condition, how they might be diagnosed (both by carer and doctor) and how they are treated.

- Urinary tract infection
- Chest infection
- Drugs
- Stroke
- Heart attack
- Severe diarrhoea/vomiting (gastroenteritis)
- Chronic skin wounds (leg ulcers and pressure sores)
- Sugar diabetes

In the very frail the following can also precipitate an acute confusional state:

- Moving house/admission to sheltered housing, old people's home or nursing home.
- Admission/discharge from hospital
- Accidental fall
- Bereavement
- Failing eyesight and hearing

Urinary tract infection

This is a very common condition, especially in elderly women. When it occurs in men it is often associated with a problem of the prostate gland, making it difficult for the man to pass water at all. There are many reasons why urinary tract infections are more common in elderly women. The short passage from the bladder to the outside means that infection can easily and quickly enter the bladder, particularly if the area between the bottom and the front passage is not kept especially clean – if a woman wipes her bottom forwards then the front passage can easily get soiled and infected. Also, as a woman gets older she produces less hormones, which results in the front passage getting dry and sore, and infection can

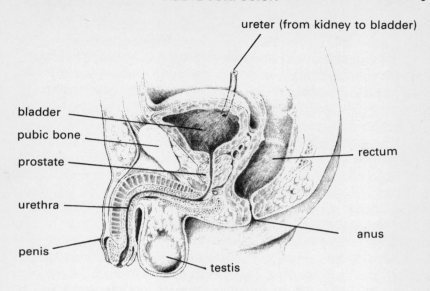

Male genitourinary system

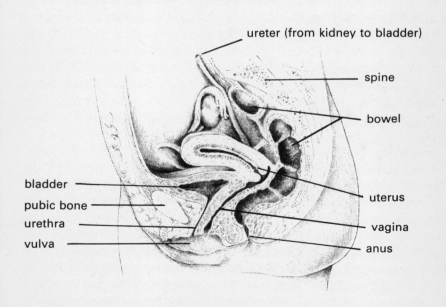

Female genitourinary system

occur more easily. Infections of all kinds occur more often if the person has sugar diabetes. Dehydration and a poor urine flow may also lead to an increased tendency to infections.

Apart from becoming confused, there are many other ways in which a urinary tract infection can show itself. The urine may smell strongly and be quite offensive. It may also hurt to pass it, causing a burning sensation or even more severe pain. Commonly it causes incontinence, in which case the infected urine can then be smelt and detected by the carers. Occasionally in a woman the infection' may be so bad as to make it impossible to pass urine; the bladder then becomes painfully full and small amounts of urine leak out. Rarely the infection causes a lot of blood in the urine.

Prevention is obviously the best cure: good hygiene may help a lot. Many people believe that a good supply of fluids, especially fruit juice, helps prevent urine infections. If the hormone lack is severe (this usually needs a simple examination of the front passage by a doctor or specialist nurse to confirm it) then some locally applied hormone cream is very effective. In most cases of established infection a short course of antibiotics will cure it. It is always helpful for the doctor to have a recent urine sample to test and send off if necessary (to grow the bugs concerned and make sure that the antibiotic given is the best one). However if the person affected has become incontinent and there are some of the other features present, it is best to start treatment as soon as possible. If the person is very unwell (toxic or unable to pass water) then admission to hospital is necessary.

Chest infection

Chest infections occur more commonly in the winter, especially if the lungs are already diseased. Smoking is the main cause of lung damage and causes the conditions of chronic bronchitis and emphysema (breathing difficulties with shortness of breath, cough and phlegm) as well as lung cancer. People with these conditions get much worse when a chest infection occurs, so smoking should be stopped at any age no matter how few cigarettes are being smoked. An elderly person's lungs may have been affected by their occupation, e.g. coal mining, or exposure to asbestos or other forms of dust. Lungs may be weakened by other chronic diseases, e.g.

asthma, operations, complications of old tuberculosis (TB) infections, or after gassing in the First World War. Even fairly healthy lungs can become infected. In particular, influenza epidemics are very dangerous for the elderly, especially if there is already a chest problem.

Chest infections can be difficult to diagnose early. It becomes easier if the confusion is accompanied by a cough, especially a fruity one, and the person can cough up phlegm. Phlegm is often coughed up normally, especially in smokers, but it is then normally white in colour. In a chest infection it becomes green or yellow and may rarely contain some blood. The infection may be accompanied by some chest pains; when these occur on breathing deeply it is suggestive of pleurisy (an inflammation of the lining of the lungs and inner chest wall). The earliest sign that a chest infection is present is often breathlessness. This may not be complained of, but carers may notice that at the beginning of the illness the person sitting at rest is breathing quite fast and shallowly.

Chest infections are either caused by bacteria or viruses. In bacterial infections antibiotics are needed to kill the bugs. Smoking should be stopped. Sometimes the infection is accompanied by wheezing and then other drugs (often in an inhaler or vapour form) are given. Coughing helps bring up the phlegm and is therefore a good thing. However, it can sometimes become exhausting and painful and needs to be lessened. People with already damaged lungs may need the help of home oxygen during a new infection, but this is always supervised at the start by a doctor. Some areas of the country have physiotherapists (part of whose job is to help clear congested lungs by tapping the chest and draining the secretions by posture) who visit people at home.

Influenza is caused by a virus. Unlike bacteria, viruses are not killed by antibiotics, so antibiotics should not be prescribed, except where complications such as added bacterial pneumonia occur. Instead, treatment is supportive and along the lines stated above. It is possible to offer some protection against influenza by having vaccination injections from the GP, and these are especially recommended in the very frail and in those people with lung damage. As with urine infections, if the condition is very bad then admission to hospital is necessary.

Drugs

Elderly people as a group are enormous consumers of drugs, not only those prescribed by doctors but also those purchased over the counter in chemists. However it is only recently that new drugs have been tried out in their research stage in clinical trials on elderly subjects. Such clinical trials are important because it is now well known that old people respond to drugs differently than the young. Drugs are broken down in the body or changed into different forms, but ultimately have to be got rid of. This can be via the kidneys, i.e. passed out in the urine, or via the liver, mixed with bile. The way in which drugs are dealt with by the body is extremely relevant because, as we age, our kidneys especially become less efficient and hence there is a risk of a drug build-up in the blood stream. If this happens the drug, instead of doing good, begins to cause harm, and one way this shows itself is by making the person confused.

The dose of the drug is therefore very important and for most old people it should be the smallest dose possible to give the desired effect. A good example of this is the heart drug Digoxin. This drug is used where the heartbeat is irregular and is going too fast. The drug slows the heart down. The usual dose for this drug in a young adult is 0.25 mg. This was found to be too strong for most elderly people and a smaller dose of 0.125 mg was made available. However even this is too much for most old people and a special dose is available 0.0625 mg, (P/G dose, i.e. paediatric/geriatric).

The time a drug takes to be eliminated from the body is called its half-life; drugs that take a long time to be eliminated are said to have a long half-life. Because an old person's kidneys are less efficient, it can be seen that those drugs with long half-lives are the most dangerous.

An example of this problem is best illustrated by the drugs known as tranquillisers and night-sedatives. One of the biggest groups are the benzodiazepines (e.g. Valium, Temazepam etc.) They are used to induce sleep and/or to make the person less anxious. They have many unwanted side-effects, including dependence, but one of the group – nitrazepam has special problems for the elderly. It has a very long half-life in some old people so that the drug gradually builds up and causes drowsiness by day, unsteadiness and a tendency to fall, as well as confusion. All sedatives and tranquillisers have the risk of inducing falls and confusion in the old and must therefore be used with great caution. Nitrazepam should not be used.

A single drug may cause confusion; a doctor prescribing five or six different drugs to an elderly patient is almost guaranteeing it! It is a feature of illness in old age that there are multiple problems, and some or all may require drug therapy. It is also true, however, that (like younger patients) elderly people do not need to stay on a specific drug for very long. Only rarely do drugs have to be given continuously and even then the dosage can usually be reduced over time. If an old person is given five or six drugs in hospital then, if at all possible, they should be down to at least three by the date of discharge. The GP can usually safely reduce them still further, only re-introducing a drug if the person should relapse. Multiple drug therapy leads to poor compliance (the drugs just don't get taken), drug interactions causing unwanted side-effects and, if not monitored, a continuation of some drugs when they are not needed. Repeat prescriptions in the elderly should be very carefully screened by GPs.

Some drugs are well known for their ability to cause confusional states in elderly people and if prescribed the person and carers should be warned to be on their guard and contact their doctor early if confusion does occur. All of the drugs used to treat Parkinson's disease can cause confusion, especially a group of drugs called anticholinesterases, e.g. benzhexol and drugs containing L-dopa. The effects of these drugs are reversible by lowering the dose or stopping the drug under the doctors advice. Steroids are very powerful drugs used for treating many conditions. These drugs must never be stopped suddenly, and so if confusion occurs a doctor must advise on the best course of action. Water-tablets (diuretics) are used in the treatment of heart-failure when there is an excess of fluid in the body. They can be gentle or very powerful but all have the potential of depleting the body of salts (sodium and potassium) and if taken for too long or in too high a dose of causing dehydration. Both side-effects can cause confusion in the old. Rarely, they are given (or taken) for the wrong reasons, such as to cause weight loss or decrease swollen ankles. They should not be used for either (swollen legs alone in the elderly is usually due to lack of mobility and the legs should be raised on a stool).

Drugs should always be implicated when a confusional state occurs. It is highly likely that all drugs can cause confusion so they must all be regarded with suspicion. When starting a drug both doctor and patient should know why the drug is being given, how long the course of treatment will be, and what are the possible side-effects. For elderly people it is a good idea for GPs to issue prescription cards listing current medication, dose and length of course. Hospital admission often results in new medication. Ideally the same drug card should be used so that both patient and GP know what new medication has been given from the day of discharge. It has been said that if all the drugs known to man were thrown into the sea, it would be a good day for mankind and a very poor one for the sea.

The following is a list of drugs (including both medical and trade names) known to cause confusion in some elderly people.

- **Painkillers/analgesics**
  DF 118/dihydrocodeine
  Fortral/pentazocine
  Co-Dydramol/dihydrocodeine + paracetamol
- **Muscle relaxants**
  Lioresal/baclofen
- **Corticosteroids/steroids**
  prednisolone (many trade names)
- **H$_2$ blockers/gastric acid reducers**
  Tagamet/cimetidine
  Zantac/ranitidine
- **Drugs used to treat Parkinson's disease**
  Artane/benzhexol
  Disipal/orphenadrine
  Madopar/levodopa + benserazide
  Sinemet/levodopa + carbidopa
  Selegiline/Eldepryl
- **Hypnotics/Sedatives**
  Dalmane/flurazepam
  Mogadon/nitrazepam
  Diazepam/Valium
  Tranxene/clorazepate potassium
  Librium/chlordiazepoxide

Alcohol
- **Diabetes mellitus**
  Insulin (various types)
  Diabinese/chlorpropamide
  Daonil/glibenclamide
  Diamicron/gliclazide
  Gilbenese/glipizide
  Rastinon/tolbutamide
  Glucophage/metformin

Stroke

To most people a 'stroke' means a sudden weakness down one side of the body due to a clot of blood in the brain. In fact there are many types of stroke. The full blown stroke, where the weakness is very obvious, can be due to a clot of blood but is most commonly due to a gradual furring-up of an important blood vessel; finally the remaining narrow passage blocks and no more blood can reach that bit of the brain. Occasionally the stroke is due to a blood vessel rupturing (like the blow-out of a car tyre) and this is usually due to a past history of high blood pressure. All of the above types of stroke happen quite quickly and can be fatal. The many who survive often take many weeks or months to recover the use of their limbs and sometimes speech.

It is now recognised that not all strokes are as major as these. In elderly people especially small strokes can occur without any great weakness of the arms or legs being noticed. It is thought that the furred-up blood vessels cause very small clots of blood to form. These small clots get carried to the brain. If big enough they can cause slight weakness of an arm or leg (or both) but this usually goes within about 24 hours. Sometimes they cause no weakness at all but make the person confused. This too often passes but as the clots recur the same thing happens again, sometimes accompanied by blackouts or falls. This condition can be difficult to diagnose unless some weakness is seen or found or the person is known to have affected blood vessels.

These repeated mini-strokes or TIA's (transient ischaemic attacks) are important for many reasons. They sometimes occur before a major stroke, and hence give a warning so that treatable causes of major strokes can be looked for. In their own right, however, they can be treated by taking a small dose of soluble aspirin a day (the aspirin makes the blood less sticky and less likely to form clots), and there are other drugs for people who cannot take aspirin for medical reasons. The repeated small strokes always cause some brain damage and if enough occur over a long time a form of dementia can be produced.

Heart attack

In this condition one or more of the blood vessels supplying the heart becomes blocked and a bit of the heart gets damaged. In a young person this is accompanied by severe pain, usually described as 'crushing', felt across the chest. The pain often goes down the left arm and up into the jaw. Because the condition is so common, most people not only recognise the symptoms in others but also in themselves when it happens. This is not always the case with elderly people. They may have chest pain but most likely they will not. This is well known and referred to as a 'silent' heart attack. It is rarely silent in other ways though. It will commonly cause a collapse and often be associated with an acute confusional state. This is why doctors do a tracing of the heartbeat – an ECG (electrocardiograph) – in acute confusion. The tracing can sometimes look normal or have old changes present, so blood is usually taken to help confirm the diagnosis. Apart from the confusion, the heart attack can also cause shortness of breath due to fluid on the lungs and abnormalities of the heart-rate (either too fast, too slow or very irregular).

Severe diarrhoea/vomiting (gastroenteritis)

All of us have experienced the unpleasantness of having diarrhoea (passing a very loose motion). It is usually a minor problem which goes within a day or two. Sometimes it is more severe and in addition to a good supply of toilet paper one needs to drink a lot of fluids. The condition may need the intervention of a doctor and perhaps some drug therapy as well. In elderly people, however, such severe diarrhoea can make them rapidly unwell. An elderly person can quickly get dehydrated (dry tongue, collapsed and thirsty) and frequently become confused. This occurs twice as fast if the diarrhoea is accompanied by vomiting, as occurs in gastro-enteritis. The actual cause of the diarrhoea may not be serious but its effects are. Most cases of diarrhoea causing confusion need hospital admission. Many old people become incontinent of their motions when they get severe diarrhoea. This had always been accepted as due to their age, until a group of GPs were asked to question their younger patients about incontinence and diarrhoea. It was found that at least 50 per cent of them had been incontinent during a bout of diarrhoea and they had been too embarrassed to mention it to their doctor. The elderly were in fact no different.

In the very frail elderly a frequent cause of diarrhoea and hence incontinence of motions is in fact constipation. The hard motion in the back passage cannot get passed. The motions back up the bowel and finally liquid motions seep past the hard blockage. If this state of affairs is reached the hard motion has to be removed (after confirmation with an examination of the back passage by a doctor or nurse). An enema may be needed, and occasionally manual removal. In the long term the bowels must be kept regular. This is best done by a combination of exercise, plenty of fluids and a high fibre diet. Constipation may make a person very uncomfortable but it is NOT a cause of confusion.

Chronic skin wounds

LEG ULCERS

Leg ulcers are very common in elderly people. There are various types (venous, arterial or mixed) but the most common form is the venous ulcer, related to underlying varicose veins. They can occur after minor injury to the ankle area and can enlarge rapidly. They are usually fairly painless and persistent pain needs expert assessment (rule out arterial ulcer). Chronic ulcers (over six months duration) need reviewing and possibly biopsying as in rare cases skin cancer can develop. Varicose veins can be treated, but usually the ulcer itself is dressed – there are as many treatments as there are doctors and nurses.

A basic rule is that chronic wounds heal best in a moist environment – hence all dressings should be in this form. This usually involves dressings called hydrocolloids, hydrogels or

alginates, ulcer coverings that soak up fluid and keep the wound
ulcer from drying out. Healing, however, is a slow process and
during that time there is a raw area of skin that is very liable to
infection. Most treatment of venous ulcers involves pressure
bandaging of some sort (over a moist wound dressing), this effectively hides the ulcer for up to a week. This is achieved by applying
layers of bandages (usually four). The bandages have to be
applied by a nurse trained in the technique. The end result should
feel very firm but not so tight as to cause pins and needles.

There are many indications that infection is occurring:
• the surrounding skin may get hot and red (cellulitis)
• there may be localised pain; or the ulcer may begin to smell
  offensive
• the wound may leak a lot of fluid which may drench the bandages, be discoloured (green/yellow) or be offensive

The infection may enter the bloodstream and cause an acute confusional state accompanied by general malaise and often fever-
ishness. Skin infections like this need antibiotics and skilled nursing.

PRESSURE SORES

These were known as bedsores or decubitis ulcers (latin:
decumbere, to lie down). Pressure sores are areas of dead skin and
underlying tissue caused by pressure blocking the blood supply to
an area of skin. They occur in elderly people who are immobile,
frail and ill, incapable of moving around unaided in bed or of
shifting their weight in a chair. Pressure sores range from redness
and blisters to deep wounds that can involve muscle and bone i.e.
life threatening. At the start of any illness in an older person attention must be turned to their pressure areas (hips, sacrum, buttocks
and heels). The first sign of damage is a red area that does not go
white when gently pressed with a finger. Incontinence and sweating make the skin moist and easier to damage. In almost all cases
they are preventable by either regular turning or special mattresses.

Once present the chronic wound is liable to infection, as with leg
ulcers, and the signs and symptoms of this are similar except that

in many cases the wound is relatively insensitive and local pain may not be a major feature. Prevention is better than cure, but once the wound is present, skilled advice is essential. A special mattress, such as an alternating pressure mattress, prevents and heals pressure sores

Sugar diabetes

The level of sugar in the blood is kept at a very precise level in the body (via insulin produced by the pancreas). In the condition known as diabetes mellitus (sugar diabetes) the body no longer controls the blood sugar level very well. Some people are severely affected and become very ill, needing insulin injections. For most people the condition is less serious but the blood sugar still needs controlling. This can be done by diet alone or diet plus tablets. Mild diabetes is more common as we age. If the blood sugar level does rise, the symptoms include increased thirst, passing more urine and a tendency to skin and urine infections. In elderly people a high blood sugar level can cause confusion as well as the secondary effect of infection. If the condition is severe enough to need treatment with tablets or insulin, then care has to be taken to ensure that the treatments do not cause the sugar level to get too low for that too is a potent cause of confusional episodes.

Moving home

The previous comments have concentrated on common medical conditions that are known to cause confusion in elderly people. It is now known however that many non-medical occurrences can have the same effect. Many old people, because of their frailty, are encouraged to seek different accommodation. This usually means either entry to sheltered housing or to an old people's home (Part III accommodation). However, moving frail old people has risks. There is an increased chance of severe illness, including acute confusional states. There is also an increased chance of the person dying shortly after the move. These aspects have been studied more closely and it seems there are some precautions we can take to lessen the risks.

The premise on which these precautions are based is that no one should move unless they really have to. There are many reasons why people do not cope in their own homes and before moving someone great care should be taken to ensure that they are not ill, or that the community services and others could not be mobilised a little more to keep the person at home. If a move is needed, one only has to think of how traumatic moving can be when young to see how major a life event it is, accompanied in elderly people by the feelings of loss of home, neighbours and friends and a sense of failure. Trauma can be minimised by following certain rules. The first is that the person concerned must want to move. Being forced to do so is asking for trouble. Many older people are frightened of the thought of so big a decision and need time and counselling by family and professionals to see the need for change. The person must then be fully involved in the move. This means seeing and approving the new accommodation and deciding on such things as what personal belongings to take, etc. Special care must be taken when a move is contemplated with anyone who has any degree of confusion, for they are particularly prone to complications. The above plan, however, is frequently not the norm. Unfortunately many moves occur at times of crisis, ending up with a frightened individual being placed in a new environment by caring people but for the wrong reasons.

Admission to hospital and subsequent discharge is another traumatic time for elderly people. As described above, the actual move and change of environment is enough in itself to trigger off a confusional episode. Add to this the reason for admission and hospitals can become dangerous places. Most people settle and recover and want to go home as soon as possible. A successful discharge depends on many factors, the most important being communication. On admission, the team looking after the person needs as much information as possible, taking it from the person concerned as well as relatives and other important sources (district nurses and home-helps etc.) In this way a picture is built up of the person in their home environment. This picture may reveal problems already present before admission, and the reason for admission to hospital itself may throw up new problems. These need to be tackled in a systematic way, with all the members of the team using their special expertise to get the person ready to return home. The patient needs to be fully involved, and very often a short visit home (a sort of trial run is arranged) to pinpoint any special areas of concern. A discharge date is then fixed, allowing patient, carers and services adequate time to prepare. Many hospitals also run check-lists to ensure that the correct type of ambulance has been booked and that such things as house keys are available. In this way most (but not all) of the dilemmas associated with discharging an elderly person home can be dealt with.

Discharge arrangements have gained a high priority in hospital procedures and now form part of most hospital 'contracts' with the purchasers (GP or health authority) of any particular service. Discharge procedures have also been formalised with the Care in the Community legislation (Chapter 8). This also means that should something go wrong with a discharge procedure the area of fault is readily identified. Minor hiccups are probably best unchallenged. More serious errors must be brought to the attention of the ward manager, not only so that the issue can be resolved and an apology given, but so that, hopefully, similar errors can be avoided. Very serious problems are best followed up by a written letter of complaint, detailing the issues and sent to the hospital customer relations department with a copy to the ward manager or consultant. This should ensure a prompt, detailed and effective reply.

Falls

Falls suffered by elderly people are the subject of numerous books. Suffice it to say that unless a good history of the fall is available, showing it was truly accidental, then a medical reason should be sought as the cause. Accidental falls though can be extremely unpleasant. The degree of physical damage is often slight but the jolt to the system can be enormous. Not only can an acute confusional state be precipitated but there can be a tremendous loss of confidence. If the fall occurred outside, the person may become house-bound. If it occurred indoors they may be frightened of moving about and use the furniture as desperate supports. Falls due to 'silent' ill-health are often accompanied by an acute confusional state. In the very old and frail, falls can be an indicator of extremely serious consequences, as in some studies many of these people have died in the following year.

Bereavement

The death of loved ones comes to us all; it is perhaps more poignant in old age to lose one's partner of a lifetime or friends who one knew at school, then through adulthood and into old age. Perhaps most distressing of all is the loss of one's own children at a time when one was beginning to depend on them more and more. Grief knows no age barriers and is as intense at eighty as it is at twenty. Bereavement is another life event coming closely on the heels of many others at this time (loss of status, money, and perhaps home and health). Most elderly people cope with bereavement naturally, but some, especially the very frail, do not, and a confusional episode can occur. In most cases it is self-limiting and is helped if the natural grieving process can occur such as saying goodbye at a funeral service. Many carers feel that elderly people should be spared the ordeal of the funeral, but in many cases the funeral is a positive experience, the need to be present and contributing is fulfilled.

Special senses

Failing vision and hearing are common in the old – so common that many people take them for granted as ageing processes. These two complaints should always be taken seriously and acted upon as soon as possible. There are numerous causes of both that are fully treatable or at least helped. Cataracts (opacities in the lens of the eye) are eminently treatable by surgical removal, even in the very old and frail. Glaucoma (failing vision due to increased pressure in the eye) needs to be diagnosed early so that eye drops or surgery can save what sight is left. Wax in the ears is the commonest cause of deafness and is easily sorted out. Deafness should be vigorously investigated and hearing aids supplied where necessary. Increasingly, hearing therapists are giving practical help and advice on the hearing disorders of the elderly. Sadly a minority of elderly people do have significantly impaired vision and hearing. The two conditions occurring together is especially disabling. The person concerned is apt to misinterpret vision and sound, rendering them very prone to confusional episodes. These risks can be lessened by maximising their existing vision and hearing as much as possible.

The person usually relates very well to their familiar environment and carers, and within reason these should not be changed. Great problems occur when such a person has to be moved or carers change. A lot of time has to then be spent patiently re-orientating the client to their new surroundings, both environmental and human.

The management of acute confusional states

General

Before diagnosis and management, the important fact of a carer recognising that something is wrong has to occur. This may be straightforward if the confusion is associated with markedly abnormal behaviour plus incontinence or other physical symptoms. It is less easy when the confusion is not severe and there are no obvious other symptoms. If an elderly person becomes confused and this is picked up by carers, medical advice should always be sought. The sufferer themselves may be reluctant to see a doctor and carers may 'not want to bother the GP' but these feelings should be overcome because the sooner the correct diagnosis is made the better the outcome.

Once the cause is found, specific treatments can be given. In the more serious cases admission to hospital may be necessary. Common causes such as urinary tract and chest infections usually respond very well to antibiotics. Confusion associated with slight strokes may take longer to respond. In addition to the specific treatment of the cause of the confusional state, there are general measures that can be undertaken both at home or in hospital. The elderly person should be cared for in a calm environment. Loud noises (frightening for anyone) should be avoided and the room should be well lit. This will help stop the sufferer misinterpreting shadows etc. and thus forming visual hallucinations. If very confused the person should have a carer present. This will lessen the person's anxieties and the carer will be able to cater to their needs (drinks, trips to the toilet etc.) If in hospital, the patient should be allocated the same nurse as often as possible to avoid frightening frequent changes of faces. A quiet, warm, well-lit room has a very calming effect on an agitated confused person. The drinking of plenty of fluids should be encouraged (water, tea and diluted squash NOT the super-concentrated sugary fizzy drinks guaranteed to make almost all old people develop sugar diabetes.) The taking of full meals for a few days is less important.

Treatments will obviously take a few days to work and during this time the elderly person may be quite agitated and distressed. Someone in this state must never be physically restrained unless they are just about to do something harmful to themself or others, then minimal force should be used to stop the action. Restraining encourages aggressive outbursts. A guiding hand and calm but firm voice works well and distracting tactics are effective. Tip-back chairs with restraining trays, cot-sides and a tying down of limbs have no place in the management of acute confusion or any other state and should be abhorred. If a person is in great danger of falling out of bed due to agitation, then the mattress should be placed on the floor. Cot-sides and tip-back chairs by increasing the agitation mean that the confused person can injure themselves very badly, defeating the desired effect.

Specific

It may be necessary to give some calming medication at the beginning of treatment when a person is excessively agitated. It is best not to use the drugs known as benzodiazepines (Valium/diazepam, Mogadon/nitrazepam, etc.) as these may have the opposite effect and, by removing all inhibitions, cause the person to be even more disturbed.

If drugs need to be used then the ones with the least side-effects should be tried first. One drug used widely in elderly people for its calming effects in confusional states is Melleril (thioridazine). It can be given in small doses, e.g. 10 mg, and the dose increased until the desired effect is achieved. This should be a lessening of agitation and not a very sleepy or stuporose person liable to fall or be incontinent because of the drowsiness. Other drugs are stronger and can cause more side-effects, though occasionally they are needed, e.g. Largactil/chlorpromazine and Haldol or Serenace/haloperidol. This latter drug can be very helpful when the confusional state is accompanied by either severe paranoia (fear of being harmed) or aggression. All of these drugs have some side-effects, the most serious being stiffness and immobility – a form of Parkinson's disease called Parkinsonism. The drugs may have to be given by injection if the person is very disturbed or is unable to take medication by mouth. Once the underlying cause has responded to treatment, the calming medication can be stopped as most people will return to normal. The medication should not be carried on just in case.

Prompt recognition by carers and prompt diagnosis and action by GPs are the cornerstones of effective treatment.

3

Chronic confusion

Chronic confusion is defined as a confusional state that lasts longer than three months. In the previous chapter we looked at the causes of confusion that do not last as long. There are many causes of chronic, long-term confusion that can be reversed or greatly helped. The main differentiation, though, is between these treatable causes and the conditions known as 'dementia'. Chapters 4 and 5 will look at the two main causes of 'dementia'.

Chronic confusional states are very important because of the reversible causes – no one should be diagnosed 'demented' until they have had a thorough screening for the treatable conditions. The diagnosis can often be very difficult and need more than one period of assessment; for example, because of the time scale involved it is often difficult for carers to pinpoint when things started to go wrong. There is no delirium, as in acute confusional states, and the problems vary with the underlying diagnosis. Memory loss and disorientation are common but often the presentation is of someone failing to cope at home. The condition 'failure to cope' should always ring alarm bells.

The following is a list of conditions which will be discussed further. Many of them are entirely reversible, some not so. An accurate diagnosis of the confusion has marked implications for both the sufferer and carers. The discussion includes diagnosis (both by carer and doctor) and treatment.

- Hypothyroidism
- Vitamin B12 and folic acid deficiency
- Syphilis
- Depression
- Head injury and brain tumour (benign and malignant)
- Normal pressure hydrocephalus
- Parkinson's disease
- Alcohol

Hypothyroidism

The thyroid gland in the neck produces the hormone thyroxine. It is the thermostat of the body and one of its regulators. It sets the level at which all the body processes run. The gland commonly fails in old age, but it tends to do so slowly so that the effects only come on gradually. As the thyroxine level falls the body slows down. The person becomes tired and slow, but as it all happens over a long period of time many people put it down to old age. Gradually the symptoms worsen. People tend to put on weight, especially around the face which gets very puffy. Everything slows up including the bowels so that constipation is a problem. Even the pulse slows down as the body adjusts to a lower level of functioning. The person commonly complains about the cold and can never get warm, and hair loss can occur from both the head and outer third of the eyebrows. If stressed (by cold weather) the sufferer can lapse into a coma. Because all of this happens over many months, if not years, it can be very difficult for carers to notice the changes. Even the family doctor, if he/she sees the person regularly, may miss it. It is the classic condition of the doctor's mother! I often see people on trains or at functions who I am certain are hypothyroid and I wonder if anyone else knows. As the disease progresses mental faculties slow down with the rest of the body so that confusion in the latter stages is common.

In its late stage the condition is readily diagnosable – the facial appearance, husky gruff voice, slow pulse and slowed reflexes – let alone the symptoms of constipation, feeling the cold, etc. A blood test confirms the diagnosis and treatment is carried out by replacing the thyroxine in a tablet form. This has to be done extremely slowly at the beginning because the body has got used to

Symptoms of hypothyroidism

dry, brittle hair

lethargy, poor memory

puffy face, lips and eyelids

dry skin

thick tongue

slow speech

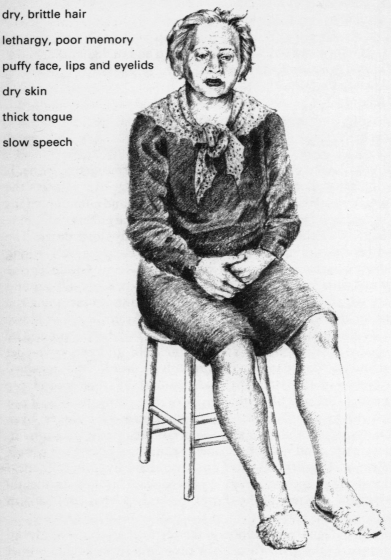

a much slower pace. Gradually the dose is increased and everything returns completely to normal.

Because many of the symptoms and signs of the condition are rather non-specific (constipation and chronic confusion occur commonly together), the blood test to check the level of thyroxine and more importantly TSH (thyroid stimulating hormone – a substance that goes up in the blood stream as the thyroxine level falls) should be given to everyone with a chronic confusional state. The thyroid replacement medication usually has to be taken for life. Hypothyroidism is especially common after the thyroid gland has been removed for overactivity when the person was younger. A thyroidectomy scar in a confused old person should always lead one to consider the diagnosis of hypothyroidism.

Vitamin B12/folic acid deficiency

These two vitamin deficiencies will be discussed together because they often coexist and have similar symptoms. Vitamin B12 is found in meat (especially liver). It combines with a substance in the stomach and is then absorbed in the small bowel where it enters the bloodstream. It is vital for healthy blood, and it is important in the nervous system. Some elderly people fail to produce the substance in the stomach which vitamin B12 needs in order to get absorbed. Also there are many people who have had part of the stomach removed (usually because of ulcers) and they too may fail to get any B12 in. (The other name for this condition is pernicious anaemia, because of its slow and debilitating onset.) Folic acid is another vitamin found especially in fresh vegetables. It too is needed for blood making and a healthy nervous system. Lack of this vitamin is usually due to a poor diet. Poor diets are probably 20 per cent ignorance and 80 per cent poverty.

The two conditions present in the same way. There are usually complaints of tiredness and lethargy. If the nervous system is affected there may be complaints of abnormal sensation in the arms and especially the legs with unsteadiness and a feeling that one is walking on cotton wool. Walking may become difficult and a gradual onset of confusion may develop. The person looks pale and is usually anaemic. They often have a pale lemon tinge to the colour of their skin. A neurological examination will often reveal many abnormalities and a blood test shows abnormally big red blood cells. All these symptoms lead the doctor to consider the diagnosis and send off more specific tests. Vitamin B12 can be measured in the blood, but as there are numerous causes, often more sophisticated tests have to be done as well. The folic acid content of red blood cells is the best blood test and this is routinely performed.

Unfortunately, vitamin B12 cannot be given by mouth as it is destroyed in the stomach. Therefore, when the diagnosis is made the treatment is by injection of B12. These are usually given every three months. The injections have to be continued for life. Folic acid deficiency is easily treated by either improving the diet generally or by giving folic acid in tablet form daily.

The longer the conditions have been present the less likely all the neurological complications will be reversed. The anaemia seems to improve well, but if established chronic confusion is present there are few reported cases of the mental state going back completely to normal.

Syphilis

Syphilis is a veneral disease that is usually sexually transmitted. The stage of the disease that can cause mental changes such as confusion occurs many years (often twenty or more) after the initial infection. The first stages may have been missed (painless lesions on the genitals and then rashes) or the infection may have been inadequately treated at the time. Any person with a chronic confusional state must have a blood test for syphilis. If it proves positive, some doctors also insist on a lumbar puncture to test the fluid in the spinal canal for syphilis as well. Sometimes the blood test is positive, indicating previous infection, but the spinal fluid (cerebrospinal fluid) is negative, showing that the infection is not causing the confusion and does not need to be treated. Some doctors do not insist on a lumbar puncture but treat according to the blood tests.

If treatment is necessary it usually consists of daily penicillin injections for about three weeks. The spouse may also have the infection and so positive cases are usually referred to the department of genito-urinary medicine so that skilled counsellors can interview relatives and explain the need for further tests on them. The sooner the infection is treated the better the results. By the time the disease has caused a confusional state, complete recovery of full mental faculties is unlikely.

Depression

Depression in the elderly is also called 'pseudo-dementia', i.e. false-dementia; this is because the symptoms and signs of depression can be very difficult to separate from those of some of the dementing illnesses. Depression is common in old age, and the elderly have the highest rate of successful suicide attempts. Depression often accompanies physical ill-health and, as we have seen before, old age is also a time of loss, making coping with the burdens of everyday life that bit more difficult.

All of us have days where we feel sad, but for most the mood passes. It becomes a problem when the melancholic outlook on life persists and begins to intrude into the person's daily activities. Common feelings in depressed people are those of worthlessness and a hopeless outlook to the future. Sleep becomes disordered and there is early morning waking with an inability to get back to sleep and a subsequent feeling of a poor night's rest. Gloomy thoughts intrude and ideas of suicide begin to form. The person may worry about their general health and consult their doctor about many trivial complaints (hypochondriasis), or they may begin to feel that their body is rotten and that they are decomposing internally. Many slow down and lose the will to do anything, even speak. The person may refuse to eat or drink and thus put their life in danger.

The condition gets confused with dementia because when various questions are asked to try and establish a diagnosis, to get an idea of orientation and memory, etc., often the person does not answer, hence scoring badly. The important difference is that the depressed person, if given enough time or if they wanted to answer, would give the correct answers; as it is though, they appear confused. Some people have a long history of depression, others have their first attack in old age. Making the diagnosis is the first step, and the sooner the better. Most people with depression do go to their GP but often do not complain of feeling low. The astute GP will realise that something is wrong and begin to ask the right questions. In difficult cases the person should be referred to a psychiatrist. There is still great stigma attached to psychiatric disease, which is odd considering that a significant proportion of the population will suffer from it during their lifetime. As psychiatric units cease to be housed in vast institutions and become part of the general hospital or community facilities, hopefully this feeling will fade. There has been a tendency for GPs to diagnose depression but be reluctant to prescribe anti-depressants for the elderly age group. This is now recognised as poor management: good clinical practice is the use of anti-depressant drugs when the diagnosis is made.

In a few the depressive illness will be part of a reaction to bereavement or disability or other stressful life events. Most of these cases will be monitored by the GP and psychiatrist and a few will need treatment with counselling. In the other cases anti-depressant drugs are needed as well as the other support networks (day hospitals, self-help groups, counselling etc.) The drugs are very effective and have minimal side-effects, except in the very old and frail. Most courses of treatment are given via the GP or on an outpatient basis. Sometimes however the condition of the person is so severe that treatment has to be started on an inpatient basis. This is certainly true when ECT (electroconvulsive therapy) is used. Many people who do not understand this form of therapy or who have never seen it given are very opposed to it. However, it is an effective, safe and necessary form of therapy in severe depression and can be life saving. A mild anaesthetic is given and one electrode on the side of the head gives a minor shock, often just enough to cause a slight twitch. The only side-effects are of mild memory loss following the ECT in some people. Most treatments (both drug and ECT) are given voluntarily. Occasionally, however, the depression is so severe that the person does not recognise that they are seriously ill and they have to be admitted compulsorily to hospital under one of the sections of the Mental Health Act. This is usually done by a social worker and the GP.

Recovery from depression can be extraordinary, although some people relapse and may need further courses of treatment. Because it is common and treatable great lengths must be taken to ensure that no one is labelled as 'demented' when in fact they are suffering from depression. Occasionally the two conditions of depression and dementia coexist; as the depression is treated the dementia does not go away but is usually noted to be less severe.

Head injury

A confusional state following a head injury must always be taken seriously as confusion can occur after the event. Head trauma can be dangerous because the injury may have caused bleeding on the surface of the brain under the bone (subdural or extradural haematoma). If the bleeding is severe it will become apparent at the time, the person becoming rapidly unwell and either going unconscious or looking as if they have had a stroke. Some bleeding is less severe at the time and the person appears to recover from the injury, only to run into problems later. The symptoms can vary from bouts of drowsiness (fluctuating consciousness) to episodic or chronic confusional states. The collection of blood is best shown up using a CT scan (computerised tomography) or MRI scan (magnetic resonance imaging) where a computerised assisted machine gives a from of X-ray picture with 'slice' views of the brain. If the collection of blood is large it should be drained by a neurosurgical operation. Recovery can be complete but does depend on the degree of damage sustained.

Brain tumour

In elderly people it is rare for brain tumours to present solely as a slowly progressive confusional state. Usually the confusion is accompanied by other symptoms and signs such as headache, weakness of the limbs (usually on one side only) and falls. Brain tumours are diagnosed in the same way as the collection of blood (CT/MRI scan). Unfortunately most brain tumours in elderly people are malignant and are secondary deposits from a main tumour growing elsewhere (e.g. lung, breast etc.) Primary brain tumours of many types do occur but the prognosis for all of them is quite poor. Most tumours respond temporarily to radiotherapy or to high-dose steroids, both of which shrink the tumour and the associated swelling to stop it pressing on other vital brain structures.

Benign (non-malignant) brain tumours are quite rare. When they are detected as part of a screening procedure for chronic confusion they can be removed, depending on their size, position and on the physical state of the person concerned.

There is debate as to whether all cases of chronic confusion should have some form of brain scan (CT scan or the more recently developed MRI – magnetic resonance imaging). If all cases of chronic confusion are screened in this way the pick-up rate for brain tumours and collections of blood is low, however the general 'cost' to the individual and the real costs to the health service are very high when a treatable cause is missed. Accurate diagnosis would also be helped. The outcome in terms of type of care, prognosis and impact on carers between a diagnosis of dementia and that of brain secondaries is very different indeed. Current resources are severely rationed, however, and until that changes it seems appropriate only to scan those people where the suspicion of a treatable or relievable cause is high, and to encourage discussion between GP, geriatrician and neurologist at every opportunity.

Normal pressure hydrocephalus

I mention this quite rare condition because it can present with a chronic confusional state, and if diagnosed early it can be treated by neurosurgery. In this condition the chambers inside the brain enlarge. The consequences are threefold: the person develops difficulty in walking (ataxia), becomes incontinent of faeces (but can also be incontinent of urine as well) and develops confusion (usually described initially as loss of short-term memory, i.e. memory for recent events). These three problems are often present in people with advanced dementia, hence the importance of recognising the problem early. The diagnosis is made on the history, examination and findings on the CT scan, as well as other complicated tests.

If discovered early the potential for recovery is good. A shunt (a long tube) is passed from the chambers in the brain (ventricles) to the blood stream or a body cavity. In this way the excess CSF (cerebrospinal fluid) is diverted and the chambers revert to their normal size. In the past the diagnosis has been made late and the results of surgery have not been good, with very little recovery in mental function and the complications of the surgery to contend

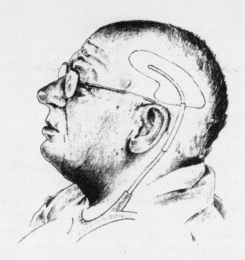

Treatment of normal pressure hydrocephalus

with. Early intervention can produce dramatic improvement and full reversal of all symptoms.

Parkinson's disease

This is a condition that most people have heard of but very few know about. It was first described by James Parkinson in 1817 and his description of his first six cases has never been bettered.

He worked as a doctor in Shoreditch in the East End of London, and whilst out in the market one day he saw two men, both were running but the front one was upright and the one behind severely stooped and only kept from falling by the front man's hand under his chin. He watched them run daily through the market area, and gradually got to know them. They were brothers, and as one became more bent over he could only stagger forwards, getting faster and faster, and would fall over without his brother's help. Parkinson made a study of the stooped brother and over the years found five other cases that he wrote up for the medical journals, describing them as having the 'shaking palsy'. His detailed assessment of the condition, later to be known as Parkinson's disease, missed very few symptoms and signs. Parkinson did however state that he thought that in this condition the intellect was spared. This is now being questioned.

Parkinson's disease is one of the most common neurological disorders of the elderly. It has many special features. One is the tremor of the fingers and hand. This usually starts on one side and is very rhythmical; the fingers are said to resemble someone who is 'pill rolling'. There is difficulty in starting a movement so that getting out of a chair or bed can be very difficult. The muscles become more stiff and rigid so that movements are slow and the face becomes blank and staring as the facial muscles become affected. All movements become disordered and the person tends to fall easily because they cannot balance well, and as the disease progresses they tend to stoop forwards and hence fall forwards. To try and prevent overbalancing the person takes little fast steps and may find themselves at a trot like Parkinson's first case.

The natural arm-swing goes, so the arms hang by the side and even the muscles in the gullet can be affected, making swallowing difficult. The skin can become very greasy with a tendency to spots, and the bladder can be affected, causing extreme urgency to pass urine and often incontinence. All these features may not occur at all in some people when the disease is very mild; for others the symptoms and signs described come on over years but can cause increasingly severe disability, all aspects of daily life can be affected, even down to handwriting, so that letters and cheque signing become impossible and buttons and laces something to avoid.

It is not surprising that depression is very common in this condition. The expressionless face and slow, often whispered, speech can lead people to think that the person behind the mask is simple. As we shall see, chronic confusion can be a feature of the condition but for most sufferers their mind is alert, seemingly trapped in a body that won't do what they want it to. The greasy skin and tendency to drool at the mouth adds to the distress and misery. Depression should always be looked for because it is amenable to treatment and can make a lot of difference to the quality of life of the person with Parkinson's disease.

Unfortunately, as the disease progresses, there is a tendency for the sufferer to become confused. At the end stages of the condition there appears to be an overlap with Alzheimer's disease and the same changes are found in the brain. For many, this intellectual

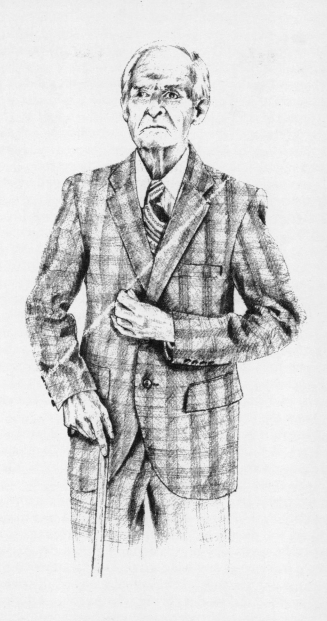

Parkinson's disease

impairment occurs at the same time as the disease stops being sensitive to drug therapy and the two systems' failures are often a terminal event. For some, however, the mental deterioration appears to occur earlier and this makes their management especially difficult. There is still debate as to whether these people are subjects with Parkinson's disease who have also developed Alzheimer's disease or whether their chronic confusion is another manifestation of the Parkinson's disease.

The latest research indicates that with Parkinson's disease, cells die in that part of the brain which governs movement (the substantia nigra, literally black area) in the brain stem (base of the brain between the ears); these dying cells form small masses called Lewy bodies – named after the man who discovered them. They are very hard to see under the microscope but are always found in the brain stem in Parkinson's disease. New techniques now mean that they can be seen more easily and they have been discovered in the main part of the brain (the cortex) in people who have Parkinson's disease and chronic confusion. The researchers feel this is a new form of dementia and have called it Cortical Lewy Body disease.

The cause of Parkinson's disease is not known. We do know that all the movement problems, and the tremor, etc., are secondary to the loss of a chemical in one part of the brain and this chemical is used to transmit the messages to the nerve and then the muscle cells. The chemical is called dopamine and is made and stored in a tiny part of the brain called the substantia nigra. We don't know what causes the chemical to disappear but symptoms don't start until at least 90 per cent of it has gone, and this probably takes many years. A picture very similar to Parkinson's disease can be caused by numerous small strokes, drugs and even Alzheimer's disease; this condition is called Parkinsonism.

The treatment of Parkinson's disease involves many different factors. Initially a lot of improvement can be gained from physiotherapy. As the disease progresses, however, it is usual for drug therapy to be used. The most commonly used drug is levodopa (contained in Sinemet and Madopar). This treatment aims to put back the missing chemical. It has revolutionised the treatment of the condition but it does not cure it; it helps control the symptoms but the disease is usually progressing underneath it all.

A comparatively new drug Selegeline (Eldepryl) appears to be valuable in treatment. It appears to enhance and protect existing levels of dopamine and is now being used early in the diagnosis of the condition. Many other drugs are used to try and control the symptoms. They all have side-effects and one of the most important is that all the drugs used to treat the condition can cause confusional states. If a person with Parkinson's disease develops confusion, the drugs they are on must always be considered as the cause.

There is no doubt that as sufferers live longer they are becoming resistant to drug treatment and physiotherapy alone, and are becoming very handicapped. Recently we have seen the exciting use of brain implantation to treat the condition. In a few centres around the world, including the UK, either foetal cells or a person's own adrenal tissue are being placed via a thin needle into the brain, hopefully to 'take' and begin producing their own dopamine. The results are eagerly awaited by doctors, sufferers and their carers, and the indications are that any benefit may take years but in some cases can be dramatic.

Cortical Lewy Body disease

It has been recognised for many years that people with Parkinson's disease may go on to develop a chronic confusional state. There was much debate as to whether this was the same person also developing Alzheimer's disease or a different condition. The breakthrough has come with better scientific techniques for looking at brain tissue under the microscope. The cause of Parkinson's disease appears to be a fall in the amount of a chemical (dopamine) produced, needed to produce normal movement, and the appearance of tiny pieces of protein within the dying brain cell – the Lewy body. Lewy bodies have until recently only been found in the same area as the dopamine producing cells, the brain stem. They are thought to be made up of various pieces of the cells' workings coming together as the cell dies.

New staining techniques have now shown these Lewy bodies to be present in the main part of the brain, the cortex (where our memory and thinking processes occur), in those patients with the confusion associated with Parkinson's disease. Researchers in the field have called this form of chronic confusion Cortical Lewy

Body disease. It appears that the disease can start as Parkinson's disease and develop into the dementia or it may start as a chronic confusional state (dementia) with Parkinsonian features developing later.

It is definitely separate from Alzheimer's disease but has some similar features. It is also thought to be very common and some researchers think it is the most common dementia after Alzheimer's disease, accounting for about 15 per cent of total cases of dementia. The dementia affects memory, language, praxis (complicated actions), gnosis (recognition of what things are) just the same as in Alzheimer's disease. There do appear to be some differences however. The cognitive impairment (all the brain functions such as memory) have a fluctuating course which does not happen in Alzheimer's disease. There are some prominent features including a marked tendency to visual and auditory hallucinations, delusions (believing a particular false idea is correct) and some aggression and depression.

This new condition may have far reaching consequences for the diagnosis of chronic confusional states. Many people with a diagnosis of Alzheimer's disease go on to develop features of Parkinson's disease. These include stiffness and some tremor. This has been put down to Parkinsonism (features of Parkinson's disease, but not all of them and hence not the true disease). It may well be that we will need to re-evaluate these people and consider the diagnosis of Cortical Lewy Body disease.

Alcohol

As many people have learnt to their cost, the effects of acute alcohol consumption can be both seen and felt. The elderly are no different in this, though their tolerance to alcohol may be diminished. Initial feelings of well-being give way to increasing loss of social inhibitions, unsteadiness, slurred speech, difficulty concentrating, then to aggressive tendencies, nausea and vomiting, and finally to falls and unconsciousness. All of the above can occur even faster if alcohol is mixed with medication. Thus alcohol abuse should be considered in all cases of acute confusional states as well as chronic ones.

Some elderly people have carried their alcohol abuse along with them for years. These are probably in a minority, for the effects of severe alcohol abuse are not compatible with a long life. However these chronic abusers may show the effects of the alcohol on every body organ. The liver may be cirrhotic (severely scarred and fibrotic) and after heavy drinking bouts they may become yellow (due to a form of hepatitis – inflammation of the liver). General nutrition is often poor and the person looks malnourished, being thin, with a poor complexion, bad teeth and skin, a tendency to bruise easily and prone to chest infections, etc. This poor nutrition can be general or more specific if vitamins are missing. Alcoholics can be deficient in the vitamin thiamine and then present fairly acutely with falls, due to an inability to walk properly (ataxia – not the acute effects of alcohol), eye problems and an acute confusional state (Korsakoff's psychosis), the whole brain condition being called Wernicke's encephalopathy. The response to being given thiamine is usually dramatic.

If the supply of alcohol is suddenly withdrawn from a chronic abuser (admission to hospital or old people's home) then it can produce the DT's (delirium tremens). This is a very dangerous condition, with a craving for alcohol and then confusion, accompanied by hallucinations. It can be fatal, especially in the more frail elderly alcohol abuser. The long-term effects of alcohol on the brain are equally as bad. Alcohol is a well recognised cause of chronic confusion or dementia. The memory loss is accompanied by a deterioration of the personality. The emotional trauma to carers is very great indeed – having to cope with a dementing person made regularly worse by bouts of heavy drinking.

Some people only turn to alcohol in late life. It may be possible to find a precipitating cause such as bereavement, depression or a chronic painful medical condition. These people usually present with frequent falls or frequent bouts of confusion that disappear after 24 hours in hospital. They have not been drinking long enough for the physical signs to show and their bodies are not dependent on the alcohol so that they rarely get the DTs. Alcohol may be smelt on the breath or found in the blood in someone who is unconscious. More commonly, empty bottles are found in the bedside cabinet during an assessment visit to an old lady who is falling over a lot, and someone has requested her admission to an institution.

Long-term dependence on alcohol is as hard to treat in elderly people as it is in the younger age groups. A commitment to stop and keep off alcohol under difficult circumstances has to be present. There are many organisations that can help but few centres for rehabilitation of alcohol abusers will consider elderly people. The late onset drinker has a better prognosis, for it may be possible to identify the cause of the drinking and treat it. There are a few people who appear to develop a drinking habit detrimental to their health after they have started to become confused with a dementing illness such as Alzheimer's disease, and these few can be particularly hard to help.

4

Alzheimer's disease

The term Alzheimer's disease refers to a condition first recognised in 1907. In that year Alois Alzheimer reported in the medical textbooks that a woman of 51 had died of 'dementia'. It wasn't the 'dementia' that caused the interest but the fact that this woman's brain had been examined under the microscope and it showed changes not seen before. In certain parts the brain fibres were tangled up and there were areas of clumping together of brain matter. As time went by, some more quite young people who had died of 'dementia' were found to have brains that showed the same abnormalities. The condition was then called Alzheimer's disease. At that time it was only described in younger people (before retirement age) and the dementia was called 'pre-senile dementia'.

It was then noted that the same type of dementia (with the same symptoms) occurred much more frequently in older people. Their brains when examined under the microscope showed the same abnormalities. Because Alzheimer had described his condition in younger people, the elderly were described as having senile dementia of the Alzheimer type or SDAT. This tended to make things rather complicated, and as dementia in younger people is quite rare it is becoming increasingly common to call the whole group Alzheimer's disease.

The two words Alzheimer's disease can't convey the complicated set of symptoms that make up the condition, unless you personally know a sufferer. A quick description often used is the slow onset of memory loss with a gradual progression to loss of judgment and changes in behaviour and temperament. A more complicated definition has been issued by the Royal College of Physicians:

> dementia is the global impairment of higher functions, including memory, the capacity to solve the problems of day to day living, the performance of learned perceptuo-motor skills*, the correct use of social skills and the control of emotional reactions, in the absence of gross clouding of consciousness.

These definitions are only guides to the whole complicated condition called Alzheimer's disease, so we need to work through some of the more common problem areas. The condition starts very slowly, so much so that close relatives and carers often do not notice that anything is wrong for a long time, then when certain things are pointed out they can often think back and realise that the dementia began a few years previously. It has been calculated that someone needs to lose about 80 per cent of their working brain cells before mild symptoms develop, i.e. problems occur late and the brain must adapt very well for a long time. It is useful to think of the condition having three phases: mild, moderate and severe – a sufferer does not always move on to the worst phase. A sudden deterioration usually means that an acute condition (such as a chest or urine infection) has occurred. A small group of sufferers do seem to have a more rapid and downwards course (like a malignant cancerous disease) and death can occur within a few years. For most however the decline is quite slow, especially if the person is well cared for and any other medical problems are tackled early and effectively. Many people with Alzheimer's die of something else (heart attack, stroke and even old age).

The most common problems are those of memory loss, disorientation, loss of judgment, changes in personality, difficulty in communicating, loss of practical skills and changes in behaviour. Thus, it can be understood that Alzheimer's disease is far more than just memory loss (as some of the definitions try to show) – eventually the condition affects all of the parts that make us an

---

* our learned responses e.g. washing, dressing, eating.

individual who relates and responds to other people. Even in the very late stages, however, a sufferer is able to show responses to kindness and gentleness, but early on part of the personality, the person's individuality, is affected. The next sections will look at some of the areas where problems arise, and later in this and other chapters practical help on how to tackle them (using basic principles) will be presented.

Memory loss

Memory loss occurs in all cases, but it can sometimes be difficult to detect as people cover it up very well. The most recent memories go first and only much later and in severe disease does the past memory get really affected. The things we've done in the last few hours, days, weeks and months are placed in our short-term memory. It is this recent storage that seems not to work properly in Alzheimer's disease. Because memory loss is an important feature of the condition and can be tested for, it forms part of every assessment. One common test is to ask the person a variety of questions covering short- and long-term memory. Ten questions are asked.

- How old are you?
- What is your date of birth?
- What is the day today?
- What month are we in?
- What year is it?
- When was the First World War?
- What is the name of the Prime Minister?
- Where are you now?
- Remember an address, e.g. 24 West Register Street and ask the person to repeat it after 5 minutes.
- Count backwards from 20 to 1.

As long as the person is cooperative (and has been asked in a nice way!) this test is easy to perform. A score out of ten is achieved. The importance of the test is that it gives a quick guide to the areas where there might be problems. The questions test short-term and long-term memory as well as orientation. A low score by itself

NEVER means that the person has dementia. It is only a guide that something is wrong. Someone with mild to moderate dementia will usually get the short-term memory questions wrong and won't be able to remember the address. They will, however, usually know their birthday (the year might prove hard) and questions about the War. The question about the Prime Minister causes a lot of debate. Mrs Thatcher was there so long and was so influential on the public in one way or another (and indeed still is) that some assessors feel it is only fair to give a point if her name is given. As a rule a low score that goes up as the weeks go by usually indicates that the initial poor performance was due to an acute confusional state. A persistently low score over many months is much more indicative of a dementia (as long as all the treatable causes of chronic confusion have been ruled out).

Psychologists are experts in the field of memory testing and use much more sophisticated tests than the modified Northwick Park test given above. When testing someone they use a whole range of different types of test so that they get a very accurate picture of where the serious memory losses are occurring. It has been shown that in mild to moderate cases of Alzheimer's dementia the sufferer can remember something (often a picture) if asked about it immediately. If the person is asked to match one picture with an identical one they can do it if shown them one immediately after the other. Problems begin to occur if a delay is introduced. Indeed after only ten seconds some people cannot match the pictures or remember what they were shown. In other tests where the psychologist tries to get the person to learn something new and then remember it, there is good evidence that a dementia sufferer can do it, can learn something new and remember it, as long as they are given long enough to do it. It seems that they forget things at the same rate as everyone else, their main problem is in learning and retaining. Computers are now being used to help test memory and other aspects that the psychologist is interested in (reaction times – the time taken for the person to press a button when asked to do so or on seeing a certain picture).

In a social setting the loss of short-term memory can be easily missed. Evasive answers to a direct question – 'It's slipped my mind', 'I'm awful with dates', 'It will come to me', are very common and it's surprising how you can start a sentence, get stuck, look at someone and they will help finish it for you. However, a stage is reached sooner or later that cannot be concealed from carers. Memory for recent events gradually gets worse and worse, whereas the sufferer can recall childhood situations and young adult life easily. This short-term memory loss can have practical implications in that kettles and ovens can be left on, etc., and people may forget that they have eaten. The sufferer may go out on an errand and a few yards out of the house have forgotten where they were going and occasionally not be able to find their way home again. In the advanced severe stage the person may forget the names of their nearest and dearest, often a very distressing state for the carers. Finally the sufferer may forget their own name.

Disorientation

Disorientation (not knowing where one is and not knowing the correct time/date/month etc.) is now being described as a very early feature of the condition. Being so closely linked with memory this is not so surprising. Usually it is the more distant things that go first, like the current year or year of one's birth. For most people it is the bit of the date of one's birthday that is used the least. Gradually the person will become muddled as to the correct month and then day of the week, etc. Getting lost outside the home does happen, but in the early stages the person can often remember their address and be got home from their expedition. Later getting lost may prove to be a recurring dilemma, especially for carers who always fear the worst in terms of accidents or illness.

Disorientation in time may take place inside the home but a person's problems with finding their way around their home rarely occurs until much later. It is well recognised amongst carers and professionals that moving someone from their usual environment can have important consequences. Sameness and continuity are very important for the confused person. They will be continent, eat, go to bed or put on the television because they are in familiar surroundings and patterns of behaviour develop. Many mentally frail people when assessed in hospital do disastrously when asked to make tea or perform other tasks. Take them home for the test and many pass with flying colours. They slot back into their routine. This is why home visits are so important before deciding on the fate of someone who is elderly and chronically confused. A sudden change of environment can not only precipitate an acute (or acute on chronic) confusional episode, it can also deprive the person of their last tentative and precarious hold on independence.

One of my patients has a moderate degree of Alzheimer's disease with poor memory and a tendency to wander. She actually managed at home with comparatively little in the way of services, having meals on wheels and an excellent home help as well as a caring family. Her family, however, found her wandering a strain as they lived an hour's drive away and would get calls from perplexed shop owners or from the police. Against advice they arranged for her to be moved to a new flat nearer them so that they could supervise her more. Unfortunately she never accepted the new place as 'home'. Every time they called she would get up with them to leave this 'funny place'. She wandered even more, and on one occasion managed to get back to her original address and persuade the local police and firemen that she had been locked out. It wasn't until they broke down the door and entered a derelict flat that they realised their mistake! Sadly she never settled and indeed was made far more dependent because she could no longer function in her new environment. The kitchen was strange and she could not remember the new way to the toilet and became incontinent. From the best motives came a personal disaster and the eventual outcome was institutional care in a long-stay unit for the elderly mentally infirm.

Keeping routines simple and regular can maintain a confused person in familiar surroundings. Reality orientation techniques are often used in institutional settings but there is no reason why the same basic format cannot be used at home. This involves the use of calendars, clocks and newspapers as well as repeating the day and month (and often clearly labelling the toilet). Visitors should be introduced by name and with an explanation of who they are.

Judgment

It is well recognised that a sufferer's judgment becomes impaired quite early on. This is especially serious when the condition affects people who are still working and when they have to make difficult, complex decisions (doctors, drivers, judges, etc.)

Obviously the person may later be at risk from being 'taken in' by unscrupulous people and can be easily made to part with money and valuables, etc. Carers may need to take on the role of financial organiser if money problems develop. Home helps frequently cash pensions for their clients, buy the groceries and help pay the bills.

Personality

Personality and general behaviour also alter with this condition. For many they are their old selves albeit with memory and orientation problems. Some however have very up and down (labile) moods. An underlying feature of the personality before the disease may come to the fore, such as a tendency to anxiety or verbal spitefulness. In the later stages underlying characteristics may become very predominant and cause problems (verbal aggression, continuing anxiety requiring continuous reassurance). Often personal hygiene becomes a particular problem, especially for carers. Washing and bathing may become infrequent (often it is forgotten) and the person may then develop marked body odour. This can be made worse if clothing is stained with urine (many sufferers appear to leave the toilet before being quite finished, hence wetting their clothes). Less time and attention is taken with wiping their bottom, leading to soiled clothing and messy hands.

Carers are particularly anxious to avoid social embarrassment as occurs with inappropriate urination or having one's bowels open in public. Undressing, accidental 'flashing' and the fondling of private parts are the other dreaded occurrences. In fact these acts do not occur often and can usually be prevented or minimised. A sense of proportion also has to be taken into account as it is not the act itself or the audience that should cause concern but the loss of dignity for the person concerned. It reminds me of a story (definitely true) that I heard recently. A rather posh woman was receiving skiing instruction as part of her expensive winter holiday. One afternoon high on the mountain with her instructor and about thirty other people she needed to pass urine quickly. She demurely approached her instructor who advised her to go behind a convenient boulder. This she did and gratefully lowered her ski pants and crouched down. Her instructor, ski party and everyone else on the mountain were thus shocked to see her bare bottom come into view and glide gracefully past them as she went backwards down the slope frantically trying to stop peeing and moving at the same time! The hot liquid had melted the snow and caused her to slide down the slope 'mooning' as she went.

As far as possible carers must try and keep their routines flexible. Some days will be better than others and it can be very difficult to keep a sense of proportion and priority. A sufferer should never be forced to try and do something but coaxed and gently persuaded. If there is refusal then if possible leave that particular task for a while and return to it later. The ideal is to tackle the problem together and not for the carer to take over. If only life were so easy!

Speech

Speech is commonly affected in Alzheimer's disease. Difficulty in finding the correct word to use is experienced early, as is the interpretation of complex conversations or proverbs and metaphors. The understanding of simple speech remains intact at this stage. Later, sentences become difficult to finish and the sufferer wanders off onto another subject and words may get repeated over and over again. Writing and reading are also affected early with word finding or spelling difficulties or a lessening of interest in the task. The taking of messages (especially over the telephone) can prove particularly difficult and may even be the situation that uncovers the early mild dementing illness.

As the disease progresses, the above communication problems steadily worsen. As the word finding deteriorates other words (paraphasias) are added in to fill the gaps so that the true sense of the communication may be lost or the wrong thing asked for. Comprehension similarly gets worse and questions may not get answered or the person may withdraw from talking altogether. Keeping a sentence going often proves too hard for the sufferer and the increasingly frequent change of subject means that the outcome becomes babbling or gibberish.

In advanced disease, communication may prove impossible and the sufferer is often unable to let even their basic needs be known. In a few people there may be an automatic verbal response occasionally, but at this stage the brunt of communicating falls on carers who will need to approach the sufferer with non-verbal means (expression, touch, etc.) Massage and stroking can convey caring probably better than the spoken word.

Dressing and feeding

Other activities can be similarly affected. Difficulty may be experienced dressing, feeding, washing and in doing other tasks. The term for this is dyspraxia. Dressing dyspraxia is very common. It shows itself with the person putting clothes on the wrong part of the body or back to front and especially the subtle difficulty of doing up buttons.

Occasionally food problems occur, although it is only late in the disease that severe malnutrition can develop. There can be many food fads and they can be especially difficult for carers. The aim is a well balanced and varied diet, paying special attention to adequate fluid intake (especially in hot weather or when central heating is on full blast). An excellent way of taking in fluid and vitamin C is with orange juice. Fruit and vegetables provide more vitamins and some fibre, and more fibre can be obtained by eating wholemeal bread and biscuits. Refusing to eat anything or even spitting food out should always be investigated further. There can be many problems ranging from gum to teeth or denture problems and including loss of taste sensation and difficulty swallowing.

Sleep

It is said that as we get older we need less sleep. This may be true for some old people but I am convinced there is a natural distribution with some needing less, a lot needing the same and some needing more (I certainly still need 8 hours minimum – prefer 10 and find 12 wonderful!) In Alzheimer's disease the amount of sleep may not change, though many carers report that their relative appears to need a lot less sleep. What may happen however is that the sleep–wake cycle changes. It appears to reverse, meaning that people with Alzheimer's disease tend to be awake at night and sleep more during the day. In itself this doesn't matter except that where the person lives with carers or with other people nearby they can be very disruptive making noise, moving around and generally acting as if it were day. These disturbed nights can be the most exhausting aspect for carers.

As far as possible it is best to avoid the use of medication though it may become necessary. Keeping the sufferer as active as possible by day is often effective as they become marginally exhausted and sleep well at night. Many however are reluctant to be too active and also nap by day (giving the carer valuable time to do other chores). A small glass of brandy or sherry will do no harm and may lead to less disturbed nights, especially if associated with a warm drink (as long as incontinence is not a problem). Night sitting services are a boon to those lucky enough to be in an area where they are provided. The client is supervised and can be up as long as they want to, leaving the carer to get at least a few nights undisturbed sleep. It should be remembered that night cramps and painful joints may disturb sleep (as well as full bladders). For joint pains and other troublesome night aches two paracetamol can work wonders. Night leg cramps can be helped by drinking tonic water (due to its quinine content).

Inevitably however some medication is needed in order to give both parties some rest. The GP should always be consulted, but safe and effective sleeping medications include **chloral hydrate/ Noctec** (500 mg up to 1500 mg) and **chlormethiazole/Heminevrin** (one or two capsules at night). Sleeping medication is far more effective if used occasionally rather than regularly.

Sexual behaviour

Sexual behaviour can cause problems. There is no reason why a couple cannot continue any sexual relations that were occurring prior to the development of the condition as long as both parties are happy. As the sufferer becomes more disabled, sexual activity usually declines naturally and both can accept this (this occurs in many other conditions, though in some diseases it may only need to be a temporary cessation).

Difficulty may arise when the sufferer (usually a man) has a resurgence of sexual urges or a wish to continue previous relations but the wife is now unhappy about this and does not want it to happen. Usually the sufferer can be persuaded to stop the advances and often the urges wear off. However, it can be very tiring and embarrassing if it becomes a persistent problem.

In a few cases of advanced dementia both men and women may fondle, touch or actively rub their genitals/private parts. This can progress to full masturbation. As with the unwanted sexual advances towards a partner, this activity can be very distressing for carers and embarrassing for all observers. Keeping a person occupied and hence distracted may help (as well as checking that there is no local cause of irritation). Appropriate clothing can lessen the activity (trousers for women, trousers with no fly opening for men). If however the sexual activity is at a level unacceptable to the carer and the dignity of the sufferer is at stake then special help should be obtained, e.g. psychogeriatrician/ mental health for the elderly as specific medication can be tried.

Risks

All of the above changes lead to some extent to the sufferer being exposed to some risks. This is never an easy topic to discuss with carers as they quite rightly feel some responsibility and above all would like the ideal solution, a totally safe environment for their loved one. There are few ideal solutions, however, and carers need to discuss the concept of risk taking with the professionals who are asking their relative to take those risks. Some risk factors can be minimised, others (accidents, sudden illness, etc.) cannot. People with confusion still have rights and the right to be at home with acceptable risks is one of them.

Measures can be taken to minimise areas of concern, often following a home visit or after talking to carers, and difficult areas can be highlighted. Homes should be well lit, warm (with automatic heating) and no open fires or very hot surfaces such as old-style radiators. Stairs should ideally have double rails and floors should not be covered with the appropriately called slip-mats. Worn or loose carpet should be removed. Doors should be secure and lock well, with a carer/neighbour keeping a spare set of keys. Walking areas should be as uncluttered as possible so that sticks and zimmer frames do not cause a fall. Footware must fit properly. Medication should be supervised or the daily require-ments left by a carer and all other medication locked away. Appliances that may be dangerous should be disconnected unless the person is safe in using them. It is obvious that not all possible mishaps can be predicted but close liaison between all parties concerned should decrease worries considerably.

A person suffering from physical as well as mental frailty may benefit from 'one room living', the concept of all of one's living needs being supplied close together. The designated room could contain bed, commode, chair, TV/radio, be well heated and made as safe as possible.

Wandering can be a particular problem, either wandering from an elderly person's own home or from an institution. Some people wander for a reason, e.g. trying to find someone or something. Frequent reassurance or photographs may help. Aimless wandering or simply getting lost causes carers great and understandable stress. The fact is that most elderly people who wander tend not to come to any harm. A few do however: they have road accidents, serious falls, or suffer and occasionally die from exposure. As with most elderly people they are unlikely to be mugged, though obviously thefts or personal violence can occur.

There is great controversy over the concept of 'tagging' wanderers (the fitting of a small device in clothing or shoes that triggers an alarm on passing through an external door). They can sometimes be used to locate someone outside. Many people feel that tagging deprives sufferers of some of their human rights and is demeaning. My personal view is that it must never be used as a substitute for adequate staffing and general care but that in a few cases with adequate discussion and agreement there may be a place for it.

Incontinence

A very common problem accompanying Alzheimer's disease is urinary, and to a lesser extent faecal, incontinence. In most cases the person can be helped, and indeed made continent again. It is not one straightforward problem, though – there are many causes and as many treatments.

It is helpful to look at the problem as being either voluntary or involuntary; that is to say the person either knows that they want to pass urine or faeces (and then doesn't do it in the right place) or the person is unaware that they are incontinent. The following list outlines the main causes of both conditions, with reference to both urine and faeces:

- Voluntary incontinence of urine.
    Immobility.
    Confusion.
    Environment.
    Culture.
- Voluntary incontinence of faeces.
    Immobility.
    Environment.
    Culture.
- Involuntary incontinence of urine.
    Urinary tract infection.
    Stress (muscle weakness) incontinence.
    Constipation.
    Atrophic vaginitis in women (dry and sore front passage due to hormone lack).
    Vaginal prolapse in women (womb dropping down).
    Prostate enlargement in men (swollen gland near bladder causing obstruction).
    Retention of urine (full bladder leaking slightly) due to prostate gland and constipation in men and infection and constipation in women.
    Drugs.
    Unstable bladder.
- Involuntary incontinence of faeces.
    Constipation.
    Haemorrhoids (piles).
    Rectal fissure (painful crack at the opening of the back passage).
    Rectal tumour (growths in the back passage).
    Neurological causes (loss of sensation and control in this area).
    Drugs.

Voluntary incontinence of urine

As the bladder fills with urine a stage is reached when we realise that we could pass urine if we wanted to and if it was appropriate, but at this stage it is not urgent – we can suppress this sensation, for example, when sitting in the cinema or on a bus. Some time later, however, another sensation tells us that we have to go soon. Gradually the feeling gets more urgent and painful. If stuck in a lift or tied to a chair, all of us would inevitably have to pass urine, i.e. be voluntarily incontinent. We would know what was happening, but force of circumstance would cause the incontinence.

A person with Alzheimer's disease in a strange environment will suffer this latter fate; they know that they need to go but often cannot communicate this or else can't find the toilet. The person is then either incontinent or they pass urine in an unacceptable place (sink, wastebin, etc.). Carers and others often know when the toilet is needed because the sufferer gets a little more agitated, begins to get up and wander and may clutch their private parts. Guiding them to a toilet quickly often saves the day. The environment is thus extremely important, not only for the mentally confused but also the other main group that are prone to voluntary incontinence, the immobile. A person with a physical handicap (such as a stroke) will find the stairs up to or down to a public toilet as daunting as you or I would find climbing Everest. A poorly designed environment can mean misery to the disabled and a lot of bladder discomfort.

Drugs (especially diuretics/water tablets) can cause sudden incontinence. The strong acting ones begin to work within minutes and fill the bladder so quickly that the incontinence starts before the person is really aware of it, especially if they are a little confused and perhaps slightly immobile. Some people sit on the toilet for a good few hours after taking their tablets, until the danger of incontinence has worn off. It is simpler and better to see one's doctor and change the medication.

We should perhaps remember that for millions of people passing urine when and where they like is a fact of life and as culturally accepted as our use of toilets with all mod cons.

Causes of incontinence in women

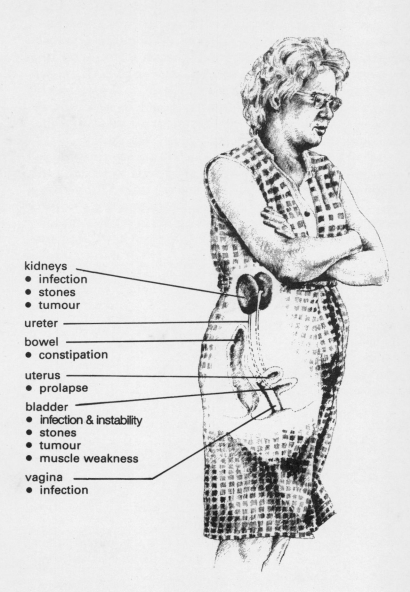

kidneys
- infection
- stones
- tumour

ureter

bowel
- constipation

uterus
- prolapse

bladder
- infection & instability
- stones
- tumour
- muscle weakness

vagina
- infection

Causes of incontinence in men

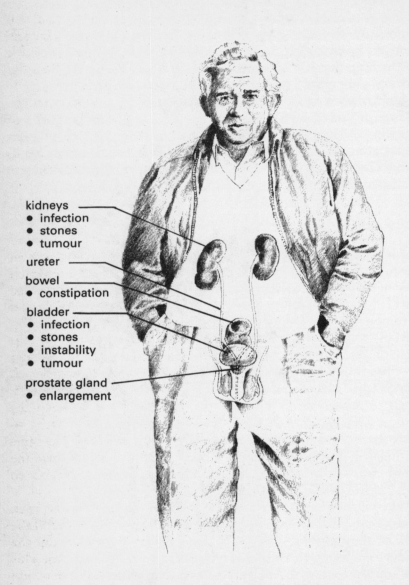

kidneys
- infection
- stones
- tumour

ureter

bowel
- constipation

bladder
- infection
- stones
- instability
- tumour

prostate gland
- enlargement

Voluntary incontinence of faeces

This is much less common, but the same basic principles as above apply. It is easy enough to ignore the desire to have one's bowels open, and eventually the urge can go away (the motions move back up the large bowel). However if this is done frequently then the motions dam up and get passed involuntarily (see below).

Confusion is again one of the main causes of voluntary incontinence of faeces, and being able to find a toilet the best way of treating it. Thus the environment and immobility also play an important role. Again, cultural differences spring to mind, for in some countries faeces form the basis of manure in the fields and are passed accordingly.

Involuntary incontinence of urine

The most common cause of this, especially in elderly women, is an infection in the urine (see Chapter 2). Severe or repeated infection may mean that the infection goes further up the urinary tract (to the bladder or kidneys) or that there is some abnormality (stones or tumour) in the bladder or kidneys themselves.

Many women suffer from stress or urge incontinence. This is often the result of childbirth, where the muscles around the bladder have been stretched and so cannot keep the opening tightly closed. Usually this means that the person wets themself if they cough, laugh or strain (and overcome the muscles trying to keep the bladder opening closed). Some women however have muscles so weak that they wet themselves soon after they stand up. The same weakness can cause a prolapse, where in its most severe form the womb drops down and can be seen. Usually the prolapse is not so bad, but still causes incontinence.

When constipation is a problem the hard motions in the back passage can push against the bladder and make it pass water. If the bulk of the motions is very big, then the pressure can stop the bladder emptying at all and the bladder fills up (retention). This can happen acutely and be very painful and needs the obstruction removing quickly. Occasionally it happens more slowly and the full bladder keeps going by emptying a little all the time, i.e. the person leaks urine almost continuously. This is a big problem in men because the prostate gland sits at the bottom of the bladder and it commonly gets bigger as men get older. A stage is reached where it begins to cause symptoms (passing small amounts of water frequently and with difficulty) and then it can block off the exit to the bladder in the same way as being very constipated can – indeed constipation and a large prostate gland in men is asking for trouble.

A woman's vagina (front passage) and the tube (urethra) leading up to and just into the bladder is covered by a delicate lining that needs female hormones to keep it moist and supple. In some women after the menopause (change of life) the hormone levels drop so low that the lining becomes dry and painful and more liable to infections. The bladder opening is also affected and the woman can then become incontinent of urine. The application of hormone creams or the taking of hormone tablets relieves this condition (see Chapter 2).

Another common cause of incontinence of urine is known as the unstable bladder. As described before, our bladders fill up with urine and as they do so we receive messages telling us how full it is. Within limits, only when we are ready do all the openings relax and the bladder contracts, pushing out the urine. All these actions take place because the nerves around the bladder, etc., use chemical messengers to tell the muscles to relax and contract. In the unstable bladder these chemicals are at fault and the bladder begins to contract when it has only a smallish quantity of urine in it and before it has told the brain it is ready – indeed, before the person is ready. The condition appears to occur more commonly in those suffering from dementia but can occur in anyone (women more than men). The classic tale is of a carer taking someone to the toilet, where they remain quite a while, then on the way out or just back in the living room the person is incontinent. It appears wilful, but is not. The condition can be diagnosed from the history and the absence of other causes, but usually a cystometrogram is done. In this test a small catheter (tube) is passed into the bladder and another one into the back passage. The bladder is filled with water and in the unstable bladder contractions of the bladder can be seen occurring too soon. Some exercises and drugs appear to help a lot, but mainly in the unconfused group who need to be able to cooperate with the treatment.

Drugs, as mentioned before, can put a great strain on the bladder. Diuretics (water tablets) especially are the main culprits. They can be either strong or weak; the most common include:

- Strong diuretics
  frusemide/Frumil/Frusene
  bumetamide/Burinex, Burinex K
- Weak diuretics
  bendrofluazide/Aprinox, Berkozide, Centyl
  Dyazide, Moduretic (not recommended by the author)

Involuntary incontinence of faeces

This is always a serious problem, not only because it is so unpleasant for both sufferer and carer but also because in most cases it is treatable but this is not realised. By far and away the most common cause is constipation. This is true whether or not the person has been incontinent of solid motion or of more liquid stools. If someone doesn't open their bowels for a long time the motion in the back passage can get very hard and it can dam back a long way, so much so that it can reach that part of the bowel where the motions are still liquid. This liquid motion then runs down the outside of the hard stool and leaks out as diarrhoea. If the constipation is very bad the hard motion pushes down and keeps the anus open so that both solid and liquid stools keep being passed. At this stage the bowels must first be cleared with enemas or manually, and then a regular bowel habit arranged.

There may be a reason why the person has been trying not to open their bowels (apart from confusion and not finding a toilet). That is why when faecal incontinence occurs, all people must have their back passage examined by a doctor – a rectal examination, quick and straightforward. There may be a painful condition obvious, such as piles (haemorrhoids) or a fissure. In the latter condition a small crack appears at the opening of the back passage, it gets inflamed and then causes a lot of pain when a motion is passed; it can be helped with creams but often needs a small operation to cure it.

Sometimes the examination will reveal a growth in the back passage. These are often painless and cause trouble late in their development. In the early stages they may bleed a little or cause constipation and then diarrhoea intermittently. If they cause faecal incontinence it is usually at a late stage. All growths in the back passage must be biopsied (a small piece of tumour taken for laboratory examination) and analysed under the microscope to see if it is a cancer or not.

Drugs can also cause faecal incontinence. Liquid paraffin is still used as a softener and laxative, but the paraffin can leak out of the back passage and cause incontinence. Some laxatives stimulate the bowel and can be quite strong, causing colic and the sudden passage of a stool and hence incontinence, e.g. senna preparations. Diarrhoea is a potent cause of faecal incontinence because the person may get very little warning and be unable to hold on to the liquid. The following drugs are well recognised causes of loose motions:

- Iron preparations
- Laxatives
- Antibiotics
- White stomach medicine (magnesium hydroxide)

If none of the above conditions are found to be the cause of the faecal incontinence then the person should be seen by a specialist as there are some neurological causes that may respond to treatment. Specialised investigations are often performed and treatment plans given. Faecal incontinence must never be accepted and put down to either age or confusion.

Incontinence aids

Following a full assessment, including toileting regimes and perhaps some behaviour therapy, there will be a residual group of men and women who need aids to help them keep dry/clean and dignified. Very few people should be faecally incontinent after a full assessment, but in severe dementia this may be the case. It is possible to constipate the sufferer with tablets, e.g. codeine phosphate, and then give them regular enemas, usually twice a week, given by the carer or a district nurse. This seems to work well with many elderly people. Alternatively pads can be used to cope with both faecal (and urinary) incontinence.

District nurses and continence advisers are the experts in the field of incontinence and should be approached to discuss all the various products available. Carers should ask their GP to arrange a meeting and an assessment.

Incontinence aids for men

Penile pouch	If the problem is occasional slight leakage.
Penile sheath	The sheath is like a condom – it stretches over the penis and is then fastened. A tube collects the urine and passes into a bag, usually strapped to the leg.
Indwelling catheter	A tube is passed via the penis into the bladder, and a small balloon on the end is inflated to keep it there. Urine drains down the tube and into a bag.
Absorbent pads	Fitted inside leak-proof pants with elasticated sides.
Absorbent sheets e.g. Kylie sheets	Placed under the person when in bed. They can be washed and reused.

Incontinence aids for women

Indwelling catheter	A tube is passed up the urethra into the bladder, and urine passes down the tube into a bag. The catheter is shorter than a male catheter and has a smaller balloon.
Absorbent pads	As for men.
Absorbent sheets	As for men.

Difficult behaviour

Unusual restlessness and agitation may indicate that something is wrong, especially in cases where verbal communication is difficult. A need to go to the toilet or another physical reason may be the cause, and should be looked for. Sometimes however it is due to the Alzheimer's disease itself, and where it becomes exhausting for both sufferer and carer medication can be given. A useful drug for this problem is Melleril/thioridazine. Wandering however is not usually the same as restlessness or repetitive behaviour, and sedating a wanderer does more harm than good, making them drowsy, unsteady on their feet and often incontinent.

Aggression by a sufferer can be very difficult to cope with, especially if persistent and severe. There are no easy answers, but the carer should not hit back, where at all possible should avoid physical confrontation and in particular should not restrain the sufferer. If it is not an isolated incident then help should be sought by asking any of the professional agencies, especially the GP. Most outbursts are triggered by a reaction, often frustration, and a subsequent similar scene can often be avoided. Persistent aggression needs specialised help from a psychogeriatrician.

Occasionally in advanced dementia sufferers bite or have other spiteful behaviour, e.g. pinching, spitting, etc. This is extremely trying and demanding for the carer, but kindness and patience usually keep the situation manageable. In order to remain kind and patient the carer needs adequate rest, occasional breaks and access to professional help when necessary.

5

Multi-infarct dementia

This form of dementia accounts for about 30 per cent of cases. It is due to repeated strokes affecting the brain. Sometimes the strokes are big enough for them to be accompanied by weakness of an arm or leg (or both), or collapse, slurred speech and facial drooping. The strokes can be fairly small, however, and cause brain damage in the form of memory loss, etc., without any of the other features of a major stroke. These multiple insults to the brain are usually due to the fact that the main arteries supplying blood to the brain are furred-up.

This furring-up process in blood vessels is known as atheroma and is more common in men. Multi-infarct dementia is therefore more often seen in men than women. Not only are the blood vessels in the brain furred up but also elsewhere such as the heart and the major blood vessels supplying the legs. It is not uncommon then for the person with this form of dementia also to have a history of previous heart attacks and pains in the legs on walking (claudication).

Following a major stroke about a third of the people recover almost completely but another third have both physical and mental impairment making them reliant on others. This first stroke can affect memory and behaviour but usually these aspects recover and it is the weakness of limbs and problems with speech that are the main handicaps. The situation changes with further strokes however. Not only does the person have to cope with any new physical disability but the brain appears to cope less well with each new insult. Recovery still occurs but a pattern develops where the person never gets back to the level before the last stroke. In this way there is step-wise deterioration.

Memory loss certainly happens and both short and longer term memory can be affected. The damage though is less global, less widespread than with Alzheimer's disease so that some areas of function in the brain may be lost while others are retained despite severe physical handicap. Because the damage is patchy, many sufferers retain insight into the problem, that is they are aware that there are parts of their memory they cannot unlock and this can obviously be extremely upsetting. The realisation of the problem can lead to some aggressive behaviour, usually simply out of frustration. As the disease progresses (i.e. as more slight strokes occur) this insight is usually lost. The brain damage can become so severe that many other problems overtake the sufferer.

Common problems

Emotions

We try to control our emotions and expression of them both consciously (one tries not to laugh at someone in the same room who is wearing a hideous hat) and unconsciously (I always cry during the last few minutes of the film *The Color Purple* even though I'm trying not to). A stroke can effectively bring one's emotions nearer the surface, lessening any control so that some sufferers cry or more rarely laugh at inappropriate times. The control system seems to be damaged. This is known as emotional lability and ranges from the person crying when a certain subject is mentioned to bursting into tears whenever they try to speak. In its severe form it is obviously very disabling both in terms of rehabilitation and socially. There is good evidence that one of the anti-depressants – amitryptiline – in a dose too low for it to be having an anti-depressant effect is helpful. I have used it many times with good success.

Incontinence

Incontinence of urine (more rarely of faeces) can occur after a single stroke but is more common as multiple strokes lead to a confused state. Often the condition is not as amenable to the measures discussed in the treatment of incontinence in the previous chapter. This is because it is often associated with more marked physical disability, making toileting difficult, and also because the nervous control of the bladder may be damaged making the achievement of continence difficult. Though one tries to avoid them, one may have to use some form of incontinent pad or consider the use of a urinary catheter when both the physical and mental results of multiple strokes are advanced.

Swallowing

Following a stroke there may be a period of time when swallowing is difficult. This usually recovers, sometimes with the aid of speech therapists, dieticians, physiotherapists and dentists. With multiple strokes (especially if they occur on both sides of the brain) the problem may develop with the other complications (incontinence, emotional lability, poor mental state etc.) The person may begin to get frequent chest infections or be seen to choke with every mouthful of food. The chestiness shows that some food particles are missing the gullet and going into the lungs because the act of swallowing has been damaged by the strokes. This often recovers as the person gets over the latest stroke, but in the later stages it can become permanent. The problem can be tackled in various ways. Following assessment it may be the case that certain types of food 'go down the right way'; these often include purees and ice-cream type consistencies. Liquids and solids tend to be swallowed only with difficulty. Solids should be mashed to a puree consistency while liquids should be thickened with agents such as Carobel. The position of the head and neck is also important. The best position is sitting upright with the head looking straight ahead (not tipped back). Liquids should fill the cup/glass near to the brim so that on drinking the head does not have to be tipped back. The speech therapist is the best person to give advice on the swallowing difficulties of stroke patients. Some people, however, are unable to swallow anything and then the decision has to be made about passing a tube into the stomach (a nasogastric tube) and feeding the person that way. This may only be a temporary measure as recovery of the swallowing reflex occurs. In some cases the impairment is permanent and most doctors advise that the naso-gastric tube be replaced by a more permanent feeding tube direct into the stomach, a gastrostomy. This is a fairly minor procedure and allows the nourishing liquid food to be pumped via the tube direct into the stomach. Once the feed is finished the tube can be disconnected and all that remains until the next feed is a small button-like attachment on the skin of the abdomen.

Physical and intellectual impairment

In any individual the symptoms and signs of their multiple strokes will vary and their degree of disability both mental and physical will differ. Some will have profound physical handicaps in the form of limb weakness and this will dominate their lives, their slight intellectual impairment being fairly irrelevant. For others the degree of physical handicap will be minimal, if present at all, if that part of the stroke has fully recovered. They may however be severely intellectually impaired with very poor memory, no concentrating power and limited learning ability. Speech may be affected (both in the ability to speak and in the ability to understand speech). Writing and reading powers can be damaged as well as the complicated processes of reasoning and decision making. This step-wise decline of both mental and physical powers can be devastating for both sufferer and carer.

Assessment and prevention

Despite the picture given above it can still be difficult distinguishing between multi-infarct and Alzheimer's dementia. The initial assessment always includes a detailed medical and personal history. In multi-infarct dementia there is often a strong family history of heart attacks and strokes, especially on the male side. The younger the age that these events occurred the more relevant they become. There may be a history of smoking and of high blood pressure (hypertension) as well as chest pains (angina) and/or leg pains (claudication). Heart attacks (myocardial infarction) and strokes (cerebrovascular accidents) may have already occurred. A step-wise decrease in mental faculties associated with other evidence of a stroke help make the diagnosis. Doctors look for the evidence of other blood vessels having furred-up (the ones in the brain don't do it alone). A score is built up of likely linked events named after the man who invented it – the Hachinski score. The higher the score the more likely the mental impairment is due to multi-infarct dementia.

From the previous discussion it can be seen that there are risk factors for multi-infarct dementia in particular and strokes in general. Smoking, high blood pressure, excess fats in the blood (hyperlipidaemia and hypercholesterolaemia), obesity and a strong family history are relative risk factors. That means that within reason one can do something about them. One can't chose one's parents and grandparents but if they died from heart attacks or strokes when young then one should go to the doctor and have a full screen performed. High blood pressure can be lowered and smoking can be stopped, blood fats controlled and weight lost.

Once the damage has been done over many years it is often difficult to remedy. Following one stroke others still occur because the underlying problem (furred blood vessels) is still there. Some conditions such as sugar diabetes (diabetes mellitus) have an increased risk of stroke occurrence. In some people it may be possible to prevent further strokes occurring. Firstly, as many risk factors as possible are treated. In some people the furred-up blood vessels can literally undergo a re-bore to stop further blood clots forming on the furred-up surface. The blood can be made less sticky by the use of various drugs. Low dose aspirin is commonly used now to try and prevent mini-strokes (transient ischaemic attacks). More rarely blood clotting is stopped by the use of the drug warfarin. There is some evidence that red wine may have a protective effect by increasing the amount of fat removed from the artery lining, the amount of red wine per day though is disputed. The Mediterranean diet appears to help, a diet rich in olive oil, garlic, vegetables and red wine!

It must be hoped that as we become healthier in terms of diet, exercise and preventative medicine, then multiple strokes and multi-infarct dementia will become much less common.

6

Where to get help

Formal networks

Formal networks is the term used to describe those services provided to help elderly people and their carers. These networks are supplied mainly by the state (although the term includes some work done by the large voluntary organisations and private schemes). The word formal is meant to indicate some degree of inflexibility and the fact that this group of people are paid for their services. Informal networks include family, friends and neighbours (and small voluntary schemes) and naturally tend to be much more flexible in their response to both general help and crisis intervention, it is also usually free.

Formal networks fall into four large groupings:

- Health authority
- Local authority
- Voluntary organisations
- Private schemes

In this chapter I will expand upon some of the headings listed above. The majority of the services will be available in all areas, but there will be some facilities that have developed locally. There may be something similar (but under a different name) in your area, so you must always enquire about services, especially if they are of a specialist nature. The GP, social services department and local library are the best places to get local information.

Health authority

- PRIMARY HEALTHCARE SERVICES
  General practitioner – independent or in a group practice – fund-holding or non-fund holding
  *District nurses
  *Specialist nurses – diabetic
                  – incontinence
                  – community psychiatric
                  – terminal/palliative care
                  – wound care (tissue viability nurse)
  Bath attendants (in some areas local authority)
  Community physiotherapist
  *Health Visitor
- HOSPITAL SERVICES
  Acute or Community NHS Trusts
  Accident and emergency – Casualty
  Inpatient beds – general and specialist
  Outpatient services – general and specialist
  Geriatric/psychogeriatric services
  (Health care of the Elderly/Psychiatry of Old Age)
  Inpatient beds
      acute
      rehabilitation
      continuing care (long stay)
      respite/holiday
  Outpatient clinics
      general
      specialist e.g. memory, wound care
      incontinence
      dental
      chiropody
  Day Hospital
  VOLUNTARY/INDEPENDENT HOSPITALS AND SERVICES
  Hospices and community terminal care support
  GP beds
  Respite/holiday beds

* May be managed by a Community Trust

Local authority

- SOCIAL SERVICES * *Note many social service functions have been devolved to the private sector, i.e. a private company provides the service.*
  Social workers/welfare assistants (community/hospital)
  Care managers
  Care in the community assessment teams
  Meals on wheels
  Home helps
  Specialist home carers – family aides
  Day centres/luncheon clubs
  Day/night sitting services
  Old people's homes (Part III accommodation)
  Homes for the elderly mentally infirm
  Incontinence laundry service
  Telephones/radios
  Community occupational therapy
  Aids and adaptations
  Specialist officers
  Holiday/respite admissions
- HOUSING
  General
  Sheltered accommodation (social service wardens)
- DSS. BENEFITS
  Attendance allowance
  Mobility allowance
  Invalid care allowance

Voluntary organisations

e.g. Citizens Advice Bureau (CAB)
  Age Concern
  Alzheimer's Disease Society
  Help the Aged
Local organised schemes including day/night sitting services, visiting/befriending groups, sheltered housing schemes and specialist services such as talking books, etc.

Private services

Residential homes   } *entry usually organised by social services, health service*
Nursing homes   } *informed if nursing home place is considered*
Housing schemes
Home nursing
Respite/holiday accommodation

Primary health care services

The general practitioner (GP) is usually the focal point of these community-based services. GPs are moving away from the old-style single-handed practice to more group work, often involving a number of doctors based in a health centre. These centres then become the base for the other primary health care workers and a focal point in the community. GPs are self-employed but come under the authority of the local Family Health Services Agency (FHSA). FHSA's are merging with the health authorities (purchasers) to become consortia. Government reforms of the NHS have encouraged certain GPs to become fund-holders. This implies a larger degree of financial autonomy and is only granted if the GPs concerned wish to apply, if their financial and patient base is big enough, and if they can demonstrate an understanding and competence of financial and management matters. It does mean that within certain restrictions the GP practice can operate more independently in a variety of ways (with the idea of benefiting the customers, i.e. patients). Running one's own budget can improve services (the government's intention). People have been worried however that patients seen as expensive would be deemed undesirable to fund-holding practices and either asked to find new GPs or get a less expensive service provision. There appears to be some evidence of this but in cases of concern the patient or carer can contact the local FHSA to discuss the matter further in confidence.

Until recently general practice was not seen as a very attractive career prospect unless working in a prosperous country area. This has now changed with new regulations requiring GPs to be specially trained. This usually takes the form of a 3 year vocational scheme, undertaken a year after qualifying and involving training in numerous specialities (children, the elderly, psychiatry etc.) A year is then spent in general practice under supervision. Increasingly many young doctors are being trained and then choose to remain in inner city areas improving the standard of health care to the population. Changes to GP's workload has resulted in fewer applicants recently and the possibility of a recruitment crisis in the speciality.

The government changes have also meant that GPs are being asked to meet certain targets (e.g. a certain number of children immunised) before full payment is given. This is meant to improve the overall standard of care. In addition, the government has insisted on the offer of an over-75 yearly screening programme. This means that every person over 75 must at least be offered a visit to check certain things: weight, blood pressure, hearing, eyesight, etc. Many GPs feel this is not a good use of their time as the pick-up rate is considered to be low. Many delegate this duty to the practice nurse and many practices do not follow up on the initial refusers.

The situation is complex and certainly not many new problems are uncovered if the government guidelines are strictly adhered to. GPs, however, are now in a position to widen the scope of the health check and include other services which may be of benefit, e.g. assessing levels of disability, depression, the possibility of abuse, etc. Good GP practices tend to offer good services, and as it is now easier to shop around and change GP, elderly customers should try and be more critical of the services on offer.

Being independent the services offered by GPs will vary. There is great debate at the moment on whether or not GPs should be allowed to advertise. I think advertising could improve the standards of many practices and give some people an element of choice, depending on the services offered. The elderly as a client group and carers looking after the old should ask a GP some fundamental questions.

Does the practice use an age/sex register?
    This allows the GP to be aware of the elderly population in the practice and develop schemes for their benefit.

Does the practice do its own house calls out of hours?
    The elderly especially need continuation of care. The use of deputising services often means inappropriate measures being taken and poor communication.

How does the practice arrange the special services for elderly people?
Who does the screening?
Is it available if you are under the age of 75?
What does it cover and include?
Does the practice follow up if you miss the first request?
  Some GPs offer well woman clinics which may welcome elderly
women. I do outpatient clinics in GPs surgeries enabling
specialist opinions to be obtained without the necessity of a trip
to hospital.

Does the practice offer regular (once every six months or year)
visits to the elderly house-bound?

Does the practice regularly review medication and give cards or
printouts of drugs being taken?
  Many practices by using the age–sex register are able to identify
the elderly in their practice and make arrangements for them to
be seen regularly.

District nurses are fully qualified nurses who have undergone
specialist community nurse training. Their job is a particularly
hard yet rewarding one. A group of nurses usually work out of a
GP practice, allowing good communication between the two
groups of professionals. Their work is extremely varied, from
tending to ulcers and wounds, supervising medication, giving
injections, helping the frail and sick in and out of bed and generally
giving them rehabilitative care and nursing attention. They are also
one of the main contact groups giving a kind word, making a quick
cup of tea and just being there.
  In many areas nurses are being less generalist and more
specialist. Thus, there are some nurses who specialise in the advice
on and treatment of diabetes. Terminal/palliative care and incontinence are other areas where nurses have become highly skilled
specialists involved in all aspects of that particular problem. Some
of the less skilled parts of nursing have been given over to other
groups such as bathing attendants. This service should be available
at least weekly, and more often if there are special problems such
as incontinence. Bathing someone involves skills of its own,
however, and these attendants perform a very special job.

Access to the nursing services is usually via the GP but direct access can be made through the district nursing headquarters, the telephone number being in the book under Health Authority.

Whatever services visit an elderly person, they and the carer should keep a note of the person's name and a telephone number where they can be contacted. The services concerned are usually very conscientious and aware of the need that is placed upon them. However, sometimes things go wrong (especially in these times of financial constraint), and then there can be nothing worse than not knowing if a service is going to appear or not. A phone call may solve the problem or at least it should afford a means of communication. If a complaint is justified, never be afraid to contact the manager concerned.

Acute hospital trust services

The hospital service has also undergone fundamental changes under the government's NHS reforms. One part of the reform is an identification of who gives the care (providers) and who buys it (purchasers). In most areas a health authority and GP fund-holders buy care in the form of contracts. The contract is the agreement between the purchaser and the provider (hospital) for a patient to be seen, or an operation to be performed for a certain agreed price. Many contracts are block contracts, i.e. it includes all work done for a whole group of patients (e.g. all new hips, all heart bypass operations or all elderly care etc.) Specialist work can still be organised but on an individual contract level. All emergency work, however, does not depend on contracts in the same sense (the charge is made to the relevant authority after the event) and hence should be and is immediate via the Accident and Emergency department. The main providers of this form of health care are acute hospitals. The reforms affected hospitals, which were granted Trust status – initially only a few, but now all in the UK. In a similar way to fund-holding GPs, hospitals have been encouraged to become Trusts once they have demonstrated to the government financial security. They are then given a greater degree of flexibility in how they function (types of service, pay rates, etc.) within certain constraints. The idea is that the providers (hospitals) compete for contracts from purchasers (health authority and GP fund-holders) by offering as low a price as possible per contract, combined with examples of good practice (better discharge planning, easy access to specialists by phone, shorter waiting times etc.) In addition to acute hospital trusts there are community and mental health trusts which provide more community based care e.g: elderly care, mental health etc. To implement these changes the government has had to spend millions of pounds on resource management. To compete, win contracts and avoid bankruptcy (essential for a hospital's survival now) the doctors, nurses and managers have had to have business training and view their service from that perspective. Some aspects of these reforms are obviously good, wasting resources has been virtually abolished. Checking on how we function and improving the system has been professionally constructive and beneficial to patients. One huge problem remains however, the NHS is still vastly underfunded. Demand continues to increase and medical and social advances continue to outstrip the budget.

The National Health Service is such a broad-based organisation that it copes with the acute accident victim at one end of a spectrum, to the chronically handicapped frail immobile person at the other. All areas have an accident and emergency department open 24 hours, basically capable of coping with anyone sent to it. Unless it is an extreme emergency however the person should have contacted their GP first. In some areas the A&E department serves as a GP clinic and this is wrong. It is wasteful of time and resources and this situation will hopefully improve as the standard of general practice improves and the awareness and education of the general public gets better.

Most access to hospital should be via the GP. In some urgent cases the admission may be via A&E and the GP is unavoidably bypassed. However, in all other cases the GP should arrange admission. This may mean talking to the hospital doctors directly or arranging for the person to be seen in an outpatient clinic. The GP has a wide range of choice and just because a person is elderly does not mean that they should automatically see a geriatrician. The problem may be very specific and the GP may feel that another specialist is necessary, e.g. a cardiologist (heart specialist).

However, geriatricians and psychogeriatricians probably offer the widest range of services available to older people. In some districts all people over the age of 65 are seen by geriatricians, in others the age varies, perhaps above 75 or 80. This is known as an age-related policy. Other districts do not operate this scheme and the geriatricians tend to see those elderly people with specific problems: this usually means the very old and frail and those with multiple medical and social problems needing all the expertise of the multidisciplinary team (a so-called appropriate referral or appropriate care service). Many hospitals try to integrate their general physician consultants and the 'care of the elderly' specialists; the exact model will vary according to location and local needs.

The services available within a unit for the elderly usually include beds in the main district general hospital, for the acute admission and sorting out of complicated medical problems. Admitting the acutely sick elderly to beds in isolated one specialty hospitals is now regarded as inappropriate and all districts should have their acute beds on the main hospital site. This means that the elderly are then able to receive all the support services they need – X-ray, specialist opinion, operating theatre, intensive care, etc. Some beds are called rehabilitation beds and are for those patients with special mobility problems (after a stroke, Parkinson's disease and those recovering after a fracture or fall).

As many elderly people present with their acute illness as an acute confusional state, some hospitals have wards with special expertise in dealing with the confused elderly person. These wards are often jointly run with a psychogeriatrician so that their expertise is available. Geriatricians and psychogeriatricians are the only consultants with continuing care beds (that is beds that the person can remain in for good). These beds are scarce and very expensive to the health service. This means that no one should be assigned a continuing care bed until everyone is certain that it is the correct course of action. Increasingly, multidisciplinary teams are forming panels to vet potential applicants so that the person in need gets the type of care exactly suited to them and their carers.

Most geriatricians and psychogeriatricians keep a few beds available for respite and holiday admissions. A respite admission is one where it is the carer who mainly benefits from the break of looking after a very disabled elderly person. Such beds should not be seen as crisis beds, for in those circumstances there is usually a medical problem underlying the crisis and the person is better in an acute bed. The respite beds are for the very medically stable clients, often admitted on a regular basis or rota system. Holiday beds fulfil the same function allowing carers a definite break once or twice a year. Again these beds are very scarce and get booked up very quickly. Access is usually via the GP, and hence the GP must be approached early so that the communication with the geriatrician can take place.

Apart from inpatient beds, the units specialising in the elderly will offer other services. These may range from the conventional outpatient clinic to specialist clinics dealing with incontinence, confusion (memory clinics) or chronic wounds. Some of these clinics offer open access and accept direct referrals from members of the public. Most however require a letter from a GP. This illustrates how important it is that the GP is aware of all the services available in his/her district.

Most units caring for the elderly will have access to a Day Hospital. These can have a medical or psychiatric bias but essentially they are units that treat the elderly on a day-patient basis with the emphasis on treatment and rehabilitation. On average a person attends twice a week for about a month or two and is then discharged. The whole multidisciplinary team work there specialising in diagnosis, treatment and rehabilitation. Because the person arrives in the morning (usually by ambulance) and stays for the day (including meals) there is a much longer period of time available for sorting out problems than is the case in outpatients and yet the person has the security of returning to their own home in the afternoon.

Voluntary/independent hospitals and services

In some districts small independent hospitals are being set up. Many have GP beds (that is beds the GPs have sole admitting rights to) and for many GPs they use these beds for admission of elderly patients either with comparatively minor medical problems or in a respite/holiday capacity. Some of the beds may also be used for the terminally ill, though increasingly these beds are in a hospice run by those with an expertise in the care of the dying.

Talking to doctors

Some patients and carers find talking to a doctor a nerve-racking experience: they often feel that they have not expressed themselves well to the clinician or conveyed their true feelings and anxieties. Doctors are being trained to see communication as a vital skill so that even where a doctor is not naturally a good communicator and the patient nervous, progress can be made. GPs are the gatekeepers to so many services and forms of help, that good and effective communication with them is essential. Hopefully most patients and GPs will have a good working relationship. In a few cases this does not happen, the fault, if present, may be on either side, but a patient or carer may be severely disadvantaged by an insensitive or blocking GP. The first way forward is always dialogue, putting the issue as openly as possible. If a service is refused or you are not happy with the answer, ask the GP to explain why such a service/treatment is not available or the reasons for a particular course of action. If the patient/carer is still not happy it may be possible to see a practice partner or ask if the practice has any mechanism for resolving disputes.

If no progress is made, discuss the problem with the FHSA. The outcome may be to change to a different practice but that is obviously not a guarantee that a particular problem will be resolved. It is worth remembering that after the initial referral from the GP, a service may not be at the behest of the doctor but of the service manager.

It is currently not possible to bypass the GP and get a hospital specialist opinion within the NHS (one can get it by going privately in most areas). Most GPs, however, are not unreasonable about organising a specialist opinion and a blank refusal without adequate explanation is unwarranted. Once under the combined care of the GP and specialist, the specialist will usually advise on the frequency of hospital visits and further tests. Having an appointment brought forward should be done via the GP. Direct contact with the specialist team is often possible but good practice and good communication means that they will report to the GP any client contact.

The art of good communication is a mutual understanding on both sides. Patient and carer should be given as much information and explanation as they need. In addition the doctor should appreciate the stresses of illness, of caring and the anxiety that both can generate.

Social services

This part of the local authority provides many of the basic essential services necessary to keep many elderly people at home. The key workers in social services are the social workers. This group of professional people either work out of a central head office or increasingly are in new neighbourhood centres where they also may work with specialists in housing, etc. Some social workers are also based in hospitals. Social workers can have unqualified staff working with them called welfare assistants.

In many ways a social worker can be seen as a person's advocate (someone who will do the best for that person, fight their battles when they are unable to do so). In many cases social workers offer advice that is then taken up by the person or their relatives. When someone is alone, however, and maybe frail, elderly or even illiterate, then it is the social worker who many turn to for practical help as well as human contact. It is obligatory that a person in hospital has access to a social worker.

Social work falls into two main areas. There is the practical side of arranging meals on wheels or a home help, or advising where to go and how to obtain benefits. Their other less publicised work involves helping individuals and families cope with bereavement, serious illness and advising with complicated dilemmas such as an elderly frail person needing to move to an old people's home. These tasks require great skill.

Most social workers possess these skills; what they don't possess is the time needed to work with the elderly and their carers. Much of their time is devoted to sorting out the horrendous problems surrounding the very young (child physical and sexual abuse) and very little time is left for elderly people, except in crisis situations. One of the main reasons for this is that there is a lot of legislation concerning the welfare of children and hence social services have a legal duty to respond. There is no such legal requirement when it comes to the old, and it is one of the scandals of our time.

Any confused elderly person and their carers should have access to a social worker. From what has been written in the previous chapters, you will realise that many confusional episodes will be treatable following medical intervention. Increased help and supervision at home may prevent an admission to hospital and a worsening of the confusional state. Some episodes of illness may take longer to recover from than others, and in some cases the acute illness will be overcome only to reveal an underlying long-term confusional state like Alzheimer's disease. In all these situations the link between the person affected, their carers and social services is vital.

The provision of and continuing attendance of a home help is probably the most important aspect of keeping a frail and/or mentally confused person at home. A more underrated service (except by the recipients) cannot be thought of. A home help's stated tasks are well known – cleaning, some washing, shopping and making light snacks. These tasks, together with the human contact they provide, mean that countless thousands of people have less lonely and more fulfilling lives. One indicator of their value is that in times of financial constraint or when their numbers are depleted by illness or holiday I have patients admitted to hospital because the lack of that service was the final straw – the home help was the only person keeping that individual from an institution.

Meals on wheels provide the elderly with one hot meal a day. In necessary cases this can be provided seven days a week, and most areas now cater for dietary needs as well as religious preferences. Some areas charge for home helps, most charge for meals on wheels.

Day centres for the elderly (and often for the elderly mentally infirm) are run by social services and provide some of the benefits of both the meals on wheels service and home helps. A hot meal is provided as well as companionship. Many provide transport and arrange day outings as well as special events within the centre such as recreational, diversional and even medical and legal support. They can cope with some disabilities but not usually incontinence or disruptive behaviour. A long wait to attend is often due to transport difficulties and the most serious failure of all is that they rarely open at weekends, the most cruel time for isolated elderly people.

The problems of some elderly people are very complicated but, often only for a relatively short period of time (just after discharge from hospital, or after a bereavement). Most districts now have a specialised group of people (sort of super home helps) trained to go into a person's home at a time of crisis, help them through it and then gradually withdraw. These can have various names – family aids, flying squad, etc. – but they are usually mobilised by social workers and only in especially difficult circumstances. They give a far more intensive input than can be provided by the usual statutory services.

Old people's homes – Part III accommodation

Old people's homes are the responsibility of the Social Services department. They are also called residential homes or Part III homes, after Part III of the National Assistance Act 1948 that set them up. Up until recently they were really the only provider of care for the frail elderly, unless the person had money and could afford a private rest home in the country or on the south coast. All this has now changed with government encouragement to social services to use private rest homes. This has led to many local authorities closing down their old people's homes, either through lack of demand (in areas with fairly affluent old people and lots of private homes) or because they are too expensive to run and it proves cheaper to place people in private homes inside or outside the area. Inevitably, this allows choice in affluent neighbourhoods and none in poorer ones.

The original concept of old people's homes was to provide the level of care that a relative could reasonably be expected to provide. This was fine until the numbers of very old and frail people began to rise. The homes were not designed for or staffed in sufficient numbers to cope with the increasing disability levels. Add to that the problems of mobility and mental confusion, as well as the lack of staff training, and there was a recipe for disaster. Many homes became feared and hated places, akin to the old workhouses – they became part of the retirement nightmare. After some scandals and much despair and unhappiness, things are beginning to change; for example, homes are being redesigned, moving away from large impersonal buildings to smaller areas of group living.

Most local authorities use a panel system for admission to their old people's homes. In many ways it implies a needs tested approach, but it does also mean that a social worker has to be allocated to the case and present their client's problems to a multidisciplinary panel. In this way those at risk of entering the home due to undetected illness will hopefully be picked up, and for others some way of caring for them at home will be arrived at by the panel. Specific questions on mobility and continence are asked of the social worker: a person must be independently mobile (using a frame is fine) and not incontinent (apart from the rare accident). They must also not be so confused as to be disruptive. This screening of prospective clients, allied with staff training on aspects of old age, mean that the quality of life for all residents is increased.

Ideally the person should visit a home before any decisions (on either side) are made, and many homes like a probationary 24–48-hour visit before the place is offered permanently. There then usually follows a month's trial to make sure the person settles in and that both sides are happy. It is vital that in this interim period neither carers nor social workers get rid of the person's original home. Some old people find that the advantages of living in a Part III home do not measure up to their expectations, and the disadvantages of their old home suddenly don't seem so bad – in short, they want to go home.

In many old people's homes staffing levels remain dangerously low. Payment for such demanding work is derisory, making recruitment difficult and training harder. Until these problems are tackled many old people will still dread the thought of entering a 'home'. In an ideal world the client and their carers should be as involved as possible in this decision; it is often made after much anguish and may well need the skilled intervention of a social worker. The elderly person should visit the home (hopefully of their choice) and meet the staff and other residents as well as seeing the rooms. Unfortunately many of our homes still have multiple occupancy and rarer still is the room with its own toilet. Carers are often riddled with guilt about the need for a home anyway, and when these other indignities are added the burden of leaving a loved one there can seem intolerable.

A client choosing an old people's home is means tested financially (differentiating him/her from a long-stay hospital bed that is free). An elderly person with no savings will lose all their pension and be handed back some pocket money. Those with assets (and they cannot be left to children in a will or given away beforehand) will have to pay the going rate per week. This again can cause some friction as many people save to leave their family something, and the thought of it all being used up through no fault of their's is especially upsetting.

A lot of research has been done in these Part III homes. Although the clients may enter continent and mobile, problems can quickly develop. Most surveys show that at least half of the residents in most homes are incontinent of urine and that at least a quarter are severely mentally confused. One way of trying to cope with these very disabled people is to adapt some homes (at least one in each district) to specialise in the care of the elderly mentally infirm (EMI). In these homes special staff-to-client ratios are needed, as well as special staff training. Reality orientation and behaviour therapy methods are used to manage difficult problems and incontinence, but some incontinence is seen as inevitable and hence is not a bar to entry or staying in the home. Other ways of helping include close liaison with the health services, ensuring good GP cover and extra input from the local geriatricians and psychogeriatricians, as well as specialised input from physiotherapists, etc.

Social services also provide the incontinent laundry service. This may just involve the collecting of soiled material and delivery of clean linen, but in some areas it also involves the distribution of pads and other incontinence devices. The laundry service is an invaluable help, and is often poorly utilised. However this service, and especially the provision of pads, etc., should only be used after the sufferer has had a full sort out of the problem, otherwise he or she may well receive the service when in fact their incontinence is treatable.

Obviously it is not possible to describe all the services that each social service department has to offer. Most are common to all areas but some services are ventures with voluntary groups and hence are only available in certain places. An increasingly important function available in some areas is that of a sitting service. This allows a carer to go out for a few hours and have time to themselves while someone sits in with the frail or confused old person. This can be a regular break or a one-off service. In some areas it is also developing into a night sitting service so that on some nights a carer can get an undisturbed night's sleep while the sitter copes with the sufferer's needs. The benefits are obvious, but there are a few drawbacks. The sitters all undergo some training (the most obvious requirement is an excess of commonsense) but occasionally the elderly person doesn't take to a stranger – a rapport has to be built up.

Telephones often form the lifeline between an elderly person and their carers and services. It is another indictment of our system that not all elderly people that need them are provided with a telephone. Increasingly the telephone is being utilised as part of an alarm system. The person carries a pendant and in times of emergency this is activated and an alarm registers in a central control room. This central area tries to ring the home (in case of accidental triggering or in the not too infrequent cases where the person wants to talk because of loneliness) but if there is no reply a car and two helpers are despatched to the person's address to take appropriate action. The peace of mind this system can give is incalculable, and yet for many there are years of waiting even to get the telephone if they need social services to pay for it.

Help in the home can be very practical as well. Community occupational therapists working from social services provide the home assessment service where aids and adaptations are needed. In cases of disability and frailty they will come and assess the person at home and provide for the changes to be made. This may include blocking up chairs to make them easier to get out of, to the provision of a new purpose-built bathroom for the disabled. They will ensure that a person's existing functions are used to the full and help them cope with new problems. If there is not just frailty but disability as well they will liaise with the disabled advisory service (again, present in most social services) for even more expert help.

In April 1993 new government legislation – Care in the Community – completely changed the way in which services were funded and in doing so set up a new assessment mechanism. The government allocated the funds for all social care requirements for elderly people to the individual districts. This money has to pay for: the home care service (home helps); meals on wheels (where it is free); residential care (local authority old people's home and private residential (rest); and nursing homes, as well as any other requirements an elderly person has (stair lift, convert bathroom to a shower unit etc.)

There is now a legal duty to assess an elderly person (at home) if they request it, or in hospital prior to discharge, and work out their individual care plan. This is agreed with the client and carer, though the carer has no legal right to insist on a service to help their caring role, one hopes they will be listened to. The care plan must then be costed. This may be simple, i.e. an old people's home charges a set amount, or a home help is needed twice a week for a total of four hours, etc. The care plans may be very complex however, including conversion costs, up to three times a day home care, telephone alarm, night sitting, etc. The care plan can only be implemented when a senior social worker, a care manager, agrees to fund the package of care.

In the hospital situation elderly people may be discharged if they require no social services or if their level of need has not changed, i.e. their care package/plan is the same. If more services are needed they have to be costed and agreed. In expensive cases the care manager will call a case conference to ensure that the high level of input is appropriate (and can be afforded by the local social services).

As with most legislation there are good and bad parts. The concept of assessment is generally welcomed, the masses of increased paperwork in preparing cost plans are reluctantly accepted. Some areas are experiencing grave difficulties, however, in two aspects. The first is the delay caused by this new bureaucracy (in most districts no new social workers were employed solely to process the assessments). The second and potentially more serious dilemma is that many social service departments insist that the government formula adopted to apportion money was seriously flawed. As a consequence some areas report insufficient funds for the care plans, hence potentially denying the elderly person their legally assessed right to a certain level of care.

The new legislation also ring fenced 85 per cent of the total monies available for the private and voluntary, i.e. the independent sector. The government is thus insisting that every social service department spends three quarters of its money on private care. Elderly people living in inner city areas therefore do very badly as these areas tend not to attract private investment and hence many people are forced into private residential and nursing homes away from their local district.

Each area was told by government to decide locally what constitutes a need for a long stay (continuing care) hospital bed and nursing home care. If an elderly person's needs are deemed a hospital responsibility then this must be provided for (and obviously this is free and a person's assets remain intact). Nursing home care has to be reported to the health authority but paid for by social services out of its care in the community budget. The difference between the two types of client can be difficult to ascertain, and as nursing-home care is means tested, i.e. an elderly person's assets (savings, house, etc.) will be taken into account to pay for the care, there is considerable interest in the decision for both client and relatives. Each area has been instructed to set up arbitration plans (for any disputes in the assessment process) and these can be explained by the care manager. The care manager is the new gatekeeper to a wide range of services, so whether it be a request for assessment of need at home, an assessment of need prior to discharge from hospital or a dispute over the assessment, its funding (or lack of), or the decision, then insist on meeting the care manager in charge of a particular care plan.

Housing

Housing is often taken for granted until a family member becomes either mentally or physically disabled. The problems associated with stairs and lifts then become very apparent. With confused elderly people the difficulties may be different. The stairs may still pose a problem but there are other areas of concern such as the person wandering out into a busy road or disturbing the neighbours by knocking on their doors. Small rooms mean that there may be difficulties with installing aids and adaptations; in contrast, many elderly people find themselves in accommodation with too many rooms after family members have moved out or died.

Private and public housing each have their own set of problems. It is no exaggeration that one should think about one's housing needs as an elderly person (perhaps with some disability) very early on, well before reaching that stage. The physical layout of the house is only one part of the equation, though. The closeness of friends and relatives is very important, especially when an informal network is needed in a crisis. Shops, parks and leisure facilities, as well as transport, all have to be taken into account (in that group of the population who have a choice over these sort of things). And there are increasing fears of break-ins and violence generally, the media especially painting a picture of the old and frail as victims; this leads to many frightened and housebound people, even though the statistics show that it is still the younger groups in society that are the most vulnerable to muggings, etc.

In the public sector, although very stretched, housing departments will do all they can to move people into more suitable accommodation – ground floor flats with a garden being the top of the wanted list, although because of the fear of break-ins and where one partner in a couple may have a tendency to wander, increasing numbers of people are choosing first floor flats with a lift. The demand for sheltered accommodation is also rising.

This term 'sheltered' means different things to different people. In some schemes the warden acts as a relative and calls in on the occupants, all of whom have alarm systems fitted to contact the warden in times of emergency. This virtually provides some form of 24-hour cover. This type of accommodation is in the minority, though, and for most people in public housing, i.e. council housing, the warden will be employed to keep an eye on things and will definitely not be available throughout a 24-hour period. This confusion in terms and roles of the warden leads many people to enter sheltered accommodation expecting (or their relatives expect) a lot of supervision.

There is no doubt that many wardens exceed their allotted hours and thus keep many elderly mentally and physically infirm people at home. Problems may surface when the warden is away and no other care group fits the bill in providing the extra services that the warden had been drawn into. So before choosing this type of warden assisted accommodation the people concerned need to know exactly what is on offer and whether or not it fits their requirements, not only at the time but also allowing for some further physical or mental deterioration.

The process involved in obtaining state benefits to which one is entitled can be lengthy and complicated. This must never stop anyone from trying – there are many people willing to help fill in the forms correctly and advise on the benefits. The books and leaflets provided by the DSS can help, but most people need extra time and explanation. Social security offices are one place to get help, but they can be pretty daunting and the staff are often very busy. Other people who will help include:

- Your own social worker or the local social services department.
- Age Concern offices.
- Citizens Advice Bureaux.
- Alzheimer's Disease Society.
- **Carers National Association.**

There are three main benefits that should not be missed if you are eligible:

- Attendance allowance
- Mobility allowance
- Invalid care allowance

Many people apply the first time without getting any advice and then get turned down. If this has happened or happens then the person must appeal and this time muster all the support they can get (GPs, paramedical staff, letters from voluntary organisations, etc.). Many appeals are then successful.

Attendance allowance

This is a weekly cash sum paid to the disabled person themselves if they need help or supervision because of either physical or mental disability. The money can be spent on anything or anyone and there are two rates, a higher rate if the person needs help day and night and a lower one for day or night attendance only. It is paid on top of any other social security benefits (including DSS residential care home payments in certain circumstances). The carer does not need to be identified.

If you claim attendance allowance you have to show that you have met the conditions about needing attention and/or super- vision for six months before the benefit can be awarded to you. A terminally ill claimant (he/she is suffering from a progressive disease and can reasonably be expected to die within six months as a result of that disease) is deemed to satisfy the conditions for the higher rate of attendance allowance and to have done so for the preceding six months. Advanced Alzheimer's disease (and other advanced dementias) fall into the category of terminal diseases.

There are special rules if a recipient is admitted to hospital or if they receive regular respite care – please check with the DSS.

Invalid care allowance

This is a weekly sum paid to carers if they are spending at least 35 hours a week looking after or supervising someone who also receives either the higher or middle rates of the care component of the disability living allowance, attendance allowance, or constant attendance allowance, in respect of industrial or war disablement. The carer must not be gainfully employed or in full-time education and not be under 16 or over 65. .

Disability living allowance (mobility and care components)

The benefits to severely disabled people were reorganised in April 1992. The disability living allowance is divided into two parts, payable at different rates. The old mobility allowance and attendance allowance for those under 65 were incorporated into this new benefit: the mobility part has been extended and replaced mobility allowance and the care component was extended and replaced attendance allowance for those under 65 years of age.

Claimants now complete extensive self-assessment claim forms and most claims are decided without any medical examination. Decision making is by an adjudication officer, not doctors as in the past. There is a right to review by a different officer and ultimately to an independent disability appeal tribunal.

The upper age for claiming either rate of the disability living allowance mobility component is normally 65. Those who are aged 65 but who have not reached 66 are able to claim if they can show that they had met the criteria and their disability had begun on the day before their 65th birthday. You cannot claim the mobility component for the first time once you have reached the age of 66, however once entitled it can be paid for life. The same age rules apply for the care component. The entry requirement to the lower level of this allowance is the 'cooking test', i.e. a person is so disabled physically or mentally that they cannot prepare a cooked meal for themselves.

The rules for all the benefits are very complicated. This should not put people off from obtaining their rightful benefits as help can be obtained (from DSS or social services to help fill the forms in). In addition a rejection should not be accepted if a genuine need is present (and the assessment process was either thought to be unfair or there was a variation on the day).

Voluntary and community groups

These are non-profit-making bodies, often funded by donations and with some central or local government top-up. For many carers they are the lifeline that the statutory services have failed to provide. They help in many ways, ranging from the advice given to carers and the setting up of carers' groups to practical help at home and emotional support and counselling.

Some groups are interested in one particular area of disability, and they then help with information on that condition relevant often to both sufferer and carer. They may also take on the local and national 'face' of the sufferers, representing their interests, especially at planning stages. Many carers and sufferers find great strength in joining a group that has others coping with the same problem. Others find that caring has been an isolating experience; on joining a carers' group they suddenly find others who have experienced the same problems and indeed overcome them. These carers' groups often organise social events – they appreciate the necessity of an evening off for those for whom free time is normally denied them.

The voluntary sector though has two unequal halves. There are the now national organisations with tight resources and the expertise to advise on benefits, financial help, etc. Then there are the very local schemes providing small-scale but none the less invaluable help – sitting services, emotional support at times of crisis such as bereavement or illness, and all carried out on a shoestring.

Finding out what is available can sometimes be difficult. Most places have a central voluntary office, called by many different names – Voluntary Service Council, Voluntary Action Group, etc. These are usually in the Yellow Pages under 'Charitable and benevolent organisations'. Other areas have a voluntary services organiser, and again this person may be found in the telephone book, or may be known by social workers, GPs, Citizens Advice Bureaux, local voluntary groups, e.g. Age Concern, Alzheimer's Disease Society, etc. Increasingly, public libraries are becoming places to get local queries answered.

Private care schemes

The last five years has seen an expansion of the private sector in terms of health care of the elderly that few would have predicted. The main reason for this rapid growth had been the government led inducements for elderly people to enter private homes, the government paying a substantial proportion of the bill via DSS board and lodging benefit. As soon as this means of payment was established by the government the huge increase in places began, with many private homes opening almost overnight. It is now big business with large companies becoming involved, as is already the case in the United States. The total cost escalated to astronomical sums (literally billions of pounds). The government's answer was the 1990 legislation, the NHS Care in the Community Act, which moved the funding decisions from the DSS (which was effectively limitless) to social services – given a yearly sum, 85 per cent of which must be spent in the independent sector. Private homes are in the same two broad groupings as the state sector, that is residential homes (similar to the local authority old people's homes) and nursing homes; some health districts have state run nursing homes or the nearest equivalent would be long-stay/continuing care wards in the local geriatric/psychogeriatric hospital.

Private residential homes are often called rest homes and some have gone back to the concept of the old people's home that was around many years ago. They like to cater for the elderly frail but genteel type of person. Many there are not even frail, they have chosen this type of care for the company and the lessening of worries about house repairs, etc. Standards will vary as will the fees, but as this type of home caters for the more articulate and well-off type of person, the standards and costs are usually high. Any form of mental illness, especially confusion, is likely to be an absolute bar to entry, as are any problems with incontinence.

The number of people wanting the type of home described above is relatively small compared to the total market for care and hence many homes have relaxed their unwritten rules to widen their potential client group. Many work on almost the same rules as State-run old people's homes, with confusion not being a bar to entry if it is not accompanied by difficult behaviour or wandering. Residents must be fully mobile (a Zimmer frame is acceptable) and continent, and must be able to care for themselves in a minimum way such as dressing and feeding without help.

Problems begin if the resident fulfils the criteria on admission but runs into difficulties later. In the State sector a great deal of effort will be expended to keep the person in the home while at the same time trying to reverse the problem that has arisen. This may involve the help of numerous people, from both health and social services. As we have seen before living in residential accommodation is not easy. In the private sector there is no in-built requirement to try and make a go of it. Some homes will be excellent and use the resources that are available, but some will simply ask the relatives to remove the person as soon as possible. The latter are the homes led by the profit motive who know they will fill the vacancy almost immediately.

Few private homes cater for the elderly mentally infirm exclusively. They too will vary from the superb to the awful. This type of home also tends to be more expensive because of higher staff to resident ratios.

Some problems are common to both private residential and private nursing homes so a lot of thought and guidance is needed before any decisions are made. The first problem is funding. For most elderly people the cost is now borne by their local social services department. Their care manager will obviously be looking for value for money and is only allowed to use a certain number of known and registered homes, which keep their prices reasonable.

If the client has assets, they will be expected to pay the full rate themselves until their capital falls to such a level that the social services will step in. Some carers are so desperate to find a home that they will meet the difference themselves, only to find that as the rates go up, as they invariably do, they can no longer meet the difference, and their relative has to leave. All these financial considerations have to be sorted out before the person moves in, especially if help is needed from the local authority. Many homes require a month's money in advance and some do not refund any should the client leave or die in this time.

The location of the home can be another problem. Many carers choose the private sector partly for the convenience of having a family member nearer to make visiting easier. Many old people still live in inner cities whilst their children have moved out to the suburbs or the country. For most old people the move out of their home is traumatic enough, but for many they have to move considerable distances either to be nearer relatives or simply to an area where the weekly costs are affordable. Circumstances change and sometimes carers have to move because of business commitments, leaving the person stranded in a totally new environment.

Most homes have some rules and regulations and these must be thoroughly checked before entry. The use of some of the client's furniture and possessions is very important, as is visiting, overnight stay facilities and the type of room available. Arrangements for medical cover need to be verified and, most importantly, the rules concerning a change in health, mobility, mental state, etc. Nothing can beat visiting a home, preferably with the elderly person concerned and getting an impression for one's self – clean rooms and communal areas with a happy atmosphere and a relaxed feel to staff and clients is what to look for.

If the home specialises in the care of the mentally frail, are there sufficient staff (some specially trained) and features such as reality orientation and reminiscence groups? Does the local psychogeriatrician take an interest in the home? What would happen if the client's mental state worsened? Finally, a key test, are the toilets and bathrooms clean and in sufficient numbers?

Nursing homes specifically cater for those people with medical/nursing needs and very few cater for the mentally confused with these problems. Nursing homes are more expensive to run and hence their charges are higher. Most nursing homes accept that as a patient worsens they will stay in the home, but some have cut-off levels of dependency and will then ask for the person to be removed. This area must be thoroughly explored before entry. A deteriorating mental state may be the cause for expulsion. Some unscrupulous homes will send patients to the local casualty department with an illness and then refuse to have them back. This means that a person may be admitted to a hospital far away from the area they originally lived in, creating problems for all concerned.

Many private rest and nursing homes now provide respite or holiday relief beds at a special weekly rate, although, like the State sector, this form of care is much sought after and tends to get booked up early. For some people it is a useful way of assessing the home for a later, more permanent stay.

From what I have said it may appear that the private sector is too much of a minefield to be looked at usefully. This is obviously not the case, by virtue of the vast numbers of people entering it daily. Within the private sector there are homes that put the health and social service equivalents to shame, and the sector as a whole does offer people a choice as to the type of accommodation they would like. Or does it? The government has chosen to put vast sums of money into private hands, rather than use the same money to improve the state sector's equivalent accommodation for this client group. At the same time there has been a decrease (in relative terms) of money available to both health and social services to spend on their long-stay accommodation, resulting in bed closures and difficulty getting staff.

The need for long-stay beds in the health sector will not go away, yet in some districts the geriatricians have been encouraged to get rid of all this type of bed because of the blossoming private sector locally. I do not see this as choice at all, both the USA and Australia have gone down this path with disastrous results. It is expensive and with few exceptions does not provide sufficient multidisciplinary care with enough expertise for the client group involved.

There will always be a role for the private sector in health and social care but not in this rapidly expanding way. If some of the money had been ploughed into the state sector, both health and social services would have come up with imaginative and bold schemes to provide choice and a spectrum of care for the frail elderly of all complexions. Geriatric medicine was born out of the neglect of the old and if we are not careful it will be rediscovered, and the wheel will be re-invented in the rest homes and nursing homes currently being filled in this country.

Private home nursing is available and there are many agencies that advertise their services. Many types of service are available, ranging from day nursing to night care, as well as skilled or semi-skilled cover. It tends to be expensive and currently agencies are charging up to £20 for one hour only, up to £10 for more than one hour for a nurse to provide general care.

Specialist private housing for elderly people is another area that is expanding rapidly. Many firms are realising, a little late perhaps, that there are a lot of elderly people with money to spend. For this group, many marketing skills are being used, advertising the advantages of moving to purpose built accommodation with the retired person in mind. Some schemes are simply based on architecture (no stairs, rails around baths, etc.); others are more like sheltered housing, with wardens employed and alarms fitted in the rooms. Other schemes envisage a sort of retirement village with all the amenities suited to the pensioner (similar, but much smaller to Sun City in the USA). Many financial packages are available to make purchase appear attractive. Thought should always be given, however, to a change in circumstances, especially if one's spouse is already disabled either physically or mentally. The nearness of medical and social help as well as family and friends is vitally important.

Other formal networks

Community psychiatric nurse
Dentist
Chiropodist
Optician
Occupational therapist
Physiotherapist
Continence advisors
Interpreter/health advocate
Day hospitals
Palliative Care nurse

Day centre
Hearing Therapist
Tissue Viability (wound care) Nurse

Community psychiatric nurse

These nurses are specially trained in psychiatry and usually in general nursing as well. They are often known as CPNs and work full-time in the community, supporting people with all types of psychiatric disorders. Some work with all age groups, some have a specific interest in elderly people. Many work from a local hospital setting and therefore liaise very closely with the psycho-geriatrician; others work out of health centres and therefore get referrals from GPs and other health care professionals.

CPNs cover the whole range of mental illness and therefore offer help and support to both sufferers of and carers of those with depression, anxiety states, schizophrenia, as well as dementia. A lot of their work involves coping with crises and then monitoring the situation to stop the same thing happening again. This means close liaison with social services and the other parts of the health service. It also means that they are only as effective as the next part of the chain. They are given great responsibility; they help ensure compliance with medication, and deal with the regular injections that some sufferers need.

Dentist

Many elderly people have poor dental health. In one large community survey 74 per cent had no natural teeth and many were wearing unsatisfactory dentures. There were numerous reports of mouth and gum disease as well as pain, and many elderly people felt embarrassed by their appearance, with dentures dropping out during conversation and eating. Most elderly people have very low expectations of their dental health, but carers who recognise a problem may find it very hard to get treatment, especially if the elderly person is additionally handicapped with confusion.

Most dental treatment is carried out by general dental practitioners. Some have a special interest in the elderly and may even be prepared to visit the person at home. If a person is in hospital with some other complaint a hospital dentist may be available. At the

Royal London Dental Hospital there is a postgraduate course dealing specifically with the elderly. In cases of difficulty the local Family Health Services Agency (FHSA) may be able to help and give the names of dentists willing to do home visits or who have a special expertise in treating the old and those with special needs (confused, people with Parkinson's, etc.) The community dental service will treat handicapped adults if they cannot arrange treatment from another source.

Chiropodist

This is a vital service for those elderly people who cannot perform their own foot care. This service is free for men and women of retirement age, but it is so overwhelmed that in many areas there are very long waiting lists. Clinics may be held in hospitals (often with an emergency day if you can get there and are prepared to wait), health centres, GPs' surgeries and in many other places. There is a community service but it is even more oversubscribed. Many people resort to going privately because they get so desperate. GPs can be asked to make the appointment or the chiropodist can be contacted directly. Transport should be provided for those that need it.

Optician

This is another important service because it is vital to keep one's eyesight as good as possible, especially if suffering from a tendency to confusion. It is also important to pick up early such conditions as cataract and glaucoma (opacities in the eye and increased pressure respectively). If glasses are needed the person may be eligible for vouchers towards the cost, and the DSS should be approached. Some opticians will visit the person at home but may charge. In cases of difficulty contact the local FHSA.

Occupational therapist

Occupational therapists specialise in assessing the handicapped of all ages and advising and teaching them and their carers on the practical ways of coping with the disability. Many specialise in the needs of elderly people. Some work in hospitals, others are employed by the local authority and work in the community. All like to visit the person at home, where they can advise on adaptations, aids and equipment, especially in the areas of dressing, washing, toileting and kitchen work. Some have had special training in dealing with the elderly mentally confused. If the person concerned is not in hospital then occupational therapists can be contacted via the social services department or general practitioner.

Physiotherapist

Physiotherapists are therapists concerned with helping mobility. They also specialise in pain relief (muscle and joint related) as well as special exercises for certain conditions (lung diseases, etc.) They work in hospitals and in the community; some specialise in the needs of elderly people where they have expertise in dealing with strokes, arthritis, unsteady walking and Parkinson's disease.

Continence advisors

These are usually nurses who have a special interest and expertise in helping with mainly urinary but also faecal incontinence. Some work in hospitals and also visit the community, others are community based. They will assess continence problems, give advice and perhaps treat some conditions. They may refer on to a specialist clinic, where they may also work, and advise the person on all the continence aids that are available. They can be contacted via the district health authority or GP.

Interpreters/health advocate

In our increasingly multicultural society there are some parts of the country with a lot of ethnic elders and their physical and mental health problems may pose special difficulties. It is very important that the health and social service professionals get the correct history so that they can help effectively. If the carer can translate there may be no problem, but if not or if it is a personal or embarrassing issue, an interpreter will be needed. In many hospitals and social service departments with large ethnic minorities to serve, there are interpreters, but they are very scarce and will need to be booked in advance if at all possible. In cases of difficulty it is best to contact the local community health council (CHC).

Day hospitals

These are run by the health authority and are either for the elderly physically frail or the elderly mentally frail, i.e. geriatric or psychogeriatric. Geriatric day hospitals incorporate the multi-disciplinary team – that means that many specialities work together including doctors, nurses, occupational therapists, physiotherapists, social workers, as well as access to dieticians, speech therapists, pharmacists, chiropodists and dentists (amongst others). The day hospital is there for investigation and treatment and should be used to save people unnecessary admission to hospital as well as acting as a place where more time can be spent supervising someone who may need special help (e.g. shortly after discharge from hospital).

The person usually attends once or twice a week (depending on the problem) for about a month or two. It is not a place where people attend over a long period but they still manage to get attached to it and the staff. Transport usually gets them there in the morning and the routine is usually tea followed by any examinations and assessments that have to be done. Lunch is followed by a short rest period and then either group work or specialist treatments, with the usually long ride home after tea again. All manner of conditions are investigated and treated and GPs should know their local day hospital well and what type of cases they can refer there.

There are usually separate day hospitals for the elderly mentally infirm. Some districts separate the day hospitals again, depending on whether the elderly person is suffering from dementia or another mental condition such as depression. Day hospitals catering for the elderly mentally infirm not only confirm the diagnosis but can try and help with any particular problems the sufferer has or the carer has noticed. This may mean helping with disordered behaviour, aggression, medication difficulties, sleep disorders and all the other problems that can occur. The two types of day hospital should liaise closely as they will have many people who will need both types of expertise, such as the problem of incontinence in the elderly confused.

Many day hospitals for the elderly mentally infirm use the technique of reality orientation therapy and in many cases will teach it to the carers. This involves telling the sufferer as often as possible about current things, especially the day, where they are, etc. Dementia sufferers especially live in the past, so this technique uses those memories as a starting point for conversation and then gently brings the person forwards to the present.

Palliative care nurse

A qualified nurse usually working as a part of a palliative (terminal care) team. They specialise in the management of terminal illness, have counselling skills and engage both client and carer. They can arrange short admissions (respites) to control symptoms or give a carer a break. They can manage and help in the last phase of life either at home or in a hospice.

Day centres

These are run by the local authority and again may be split into those that have a special expertise in dealing with elderly physically frail and the elderly mentally infirm. The idea is not for treatment and rehabilitation but for a place to go for companionship, a hot meal and a lot of diversional therapy (be it card games, outings, special talks, fund-raising drives, etc.). Carers get a break, while the person concerned usually has a very full day out. Day centres obviously vary as to their standards but most have waiting lists to get in. In many cases it is the provision of transport that is the hold-up. Some do not cater for the very physically handicapped or for those with special needs (blindness, incontinence, confusion), although there may be a centre locally specifically dealing with that minority group.

Hearing therapist

Hearing therapy is a relatively new specialty introduced to provide more continuous comprehensive help than was possible by issuing hearing aids alone. The therapist tries to help individuals with an acquired hearing loss make the most of their residual hearing, teaching them to use every available auditory and visual clue and thus making it possible for them to live with less anxieties in a world that relies on language for communication. The hearing therapist is concerned with rehabilitating the hearing impaired person, and a tailormade programme is planned which includes auditory training, lipreading, help with the hearing aid, advice on environmental aids and advice on how to cope with hearing loss.

Tissue viability (wound care) nurse

This specialist nurse is an expert in the field of chronic wounds (usually leg ulcers and pressure sores). Pressure sores can be a major problem when an elderly person becomes immobile and perhaps incontinent. Most sores can be prevented and the specialist nurse can give practical advice on the special mattresses that are available. Should a pressure sore develop they can advise on the treatment of the wound.

Informal networks

This title includes family, friends and neighbours – the carers who provide the flexible 24-hour a day help. The vast bulk of this network are women, estimated to number about 1¼ million.

The act of caring can become a burden, so much so that the carer begins to feel guilty about feelings of resentment towards the person they care for. Many excellent books have been written which analyse this role of being a carer, and they offer very practical advice on how to cope with the situation (see further reading). The need for guidance has led to the formation of organisations such as the Carers National Association, which fulfils this role.

What is evident on meeting carers of both the elderly and the elderly mentally infirm is that they all have similar problems, with personal variations, and yet many feel that they are the only carer experiencing these problems. Many carers feel angry at being put in a caring role, sometimes wanting to direct this anger at the sufferer and sometimes at other family members or professionals for not helping more. Many feel frightened at the thought of calling for help in case people see it as a sign of not caring. Some carers feel obliged to give up jobs and personal relationships, often as the result of badly thought-out professional advice. They then have to cope with feelings of resentment. Some carers are put into the dilemma of feeling they have to choose between their elderly confused relative and husband, children or perhaps their job.

Many carers get acutely embarrassed by the behaviour of their confused relative. Incontinence, eating habits or bad language can appear monumental problems, keeping the sufferer and carer alike prisoners at home. Family, friends and neighbours should be able to help by sharing some of the more exhausting aspects of caring. Voluntary and community groups can act as an information service which can result in the carer getting the counselling they need. Most importantly these groups can put carers in touch with each other and arrange meetings. It is at these meetings that carers discover how many of them have the same problems and how some have come up with answers. Many schemes organise carers' groups that not only have a much needed social role but also arrange for visiting and support. In this way carers can get specialist advice on their sufferers' problems and if necessary be directed towards extra services or professional help.

Informal networks are not the answer to every problem; in fact for many carers there are no easy answers and sometimes very difficult decisions concerning family members have to be made. The fact that so many people do care is heartening in itself, but there is a growing anger that this role is being taken for granted and that only small-scale volunteer groups are making the headway needed to help so many people. Most carers are happy to go on caring in the right circumstances given the support and advice they feel that they and their sufferer need.

The majority of our dependent elderly survive at home, both physically and mentally, because of this system of carers that make up the informal network. The strains are already enormous and if great inroads are not made into helping this group, both in financial and planning terms, then a large number of them will be forced to give up. For many obvious reasons, that would be a tragedy but perhaps cynically in our current economic climate it would also be hugely expensive. It is far more cost-effective to help the carers now than pick up the bill later.

7

Memory clinics

The National Health Service continues to lead the world in innovative ventures. In the face of increasingly overwhelming odds the NHS is trying to coordinate its services towards the elderly providing a range of care by dedicated people, usually with minimal financial backing. To be added to this range of services (inpatient, outpatient, day hospital, continence clinics, etc.) can now be added memory clinics. In 1983 the Geriatric Research Unit of University College Hospital, London, opened a memory clinic. The research work pioneered there inspired others, and many similar clinics have started, including one in my own health district of Tower Hamlets, opened by the late Dr Isobel Moyes.

It is obvious to all who deal with elderly people that the worry of developing memory loss and possibly dementia is very great indeed. Some of this worry stems from a knowledge of how the elderly mentally confused are looked after by the state. The mind's eye picture of bewildered old people dressed in food and urine stained ill-fitting clothes wandering around in the absence of trained carers is so strong because it bears an uncomfortably close association to the truth. The other aspect, though, is the ignorance surrounding the whole area of memory loss and dementia and the fact that this ignorance leads to untold worry and concern.

What is a memory clinic?

The purpose of a memory clinic is to investigate people presenting with the symptom of memory impairment and help in the early detection of all the possible causes including dementia. The original University College memory clinic accepted self referrals, referrals from carers and from all health care professionals, especially GPs. This wide access was thought necessary as concern on the part of sufferer and carer can be immense, and professional expertise currently poor at recognising this and detecting early and potentially treatable conditions. Thus a memory clinic will be of practical help to clients but it should also function as a district 'resource centre', with educational and research functions linked to all disciplines concerned in the care of the elderly mentally infirm. In this way general practitioners, district nurses and social services can have a specialist multidisciplinary centre where early referral and assessment could be the first stage. The next stage would be chosen from a spectrum of resources, such as the other expertise available within a psychogeriatric unit: counselling and informa- tion, day care, relative and volunteer support groups, day and night sitting, intermittent respite care, and later, if necessary, a permanent home in a hospital or community setting.

The different professionals available within a memory clinic will vary. A standard core of clinical psychologist, physician and psychiatrist is the norm. These professionals usually assess inde- pendently, collating their data to form a cumulative profile of the person concerned. Nursing input is helpful and social-work involvement extremely important.

The job of the clinical psychologist is to work out whether or not any memory loss is indeed present. To do this he/she will carry out numerous tests (see fig. 1). Some tests involve the naming of things, vocabulary tests and the ability to fit things together (cerebral function test). Others assess how quickly one can react to a com- mand or if one can remember something a few minutes after seeing it (Kendrick battery). Increasingly computers are being used as part of a range of tests. The computer tests provide statistical data and usually have good patient compliance, i.e., they are 'user friendly'.

A good history from the person (usually necessarily supple- mented by others) and full physical examination are needed. The physician looks for and rules out the treatable causes of memory loss. This screening will involve blood and urine tests, X-rays, ECG and possibly some form of brain scan. This part is extremely important: amongst the University College patients 8 per cent were found to have reversible causes responsible for their memory loss. The physician also attempts to subclassify those people found to be suffering from the symptoms of dementia into a disease type, either Alzheimer's disease or multi-infarct dementia (or indeed one of the other rare types). To do this the Hachinski score is used – a scoring system based on a list of symptoms and signs due to hardening of the arteries. A score of 7 or more usually indicates that the condition is due to furred-up blood vessels and multi-infarct dementia. The truth of the matter, using the evidence obtained during post-mortems (detailed examination of the body after death including examination of slices of the brain under the microscope), however, is that there is considerable overlap between the two conditions.

The psychiatrist in the team assesses the mental state. If any dementia is found the psychiatrist tries to work out how severe the condition is, i.e. what stage the dementia has reached. The psychiatrist also has to examine for so-called affective disorders, the most important of which is depression. This assessment will involve a fairly lengthy interview. Amongst the University College patients, 10 per cent of them were found to have an affective disorder.

At the end of all the interviews and assessments (often spanning a period of time) everyone gets together to pool their information and the people seen are placed under various headings. There will be those with no memory loss shown and hence no clinical diagnosis given. These patients can be reassured. They or their carers thought that they were losing their memory or becoming demented and the worry probably made the situation very much worse. The problem usually goes after the reassurance. Other subgroups will be found to have potentially reversible conditions or affective disorders such as depression causing their memory loss. These people are told of the possible problem and referred to their own family doctor or specialist after consultation with the GP. They can obviously be reassessed after the appropriate treatment.

There will be some people who are on the borderline of having significant memory loss. This group of people can be monitored over a period of time; definite evidence of memory loss will emerge in some (in the absence of other reasons) and the diagnosis of dementia can be made. Within this group (and they do not proceed on to dementia) are those people with benign 'senile' forgetfulness. In this condition there is the intermittent but often frequent inability to remember names, unimportant events and the location of things. A good portrayal of someone with the condition is the Margaret Rutherford character in the film *The VIPs*. In such people there are no major memory or other defects when formal testing is performed.

The last major grouping will be those in which there is clear evidence of memory loss, often with support of behaviour changes (from carers or direct observation). There may be some insight on the part of the sufferer into the problem (especially in multi-infarct dementia). In addition to memory loss the dementias can also produce other impairments and these too are assessed; examples include difficulty naming objects or finding the right word, failure to understand a written or spoken sentence, trouble dressing, not knowing which bits of clothing go where, emotional lability and personality deterioration.

The memory clinic should not just act as the place where a diagnosis is made – that is only a small part of its role. Following diagnosis there should be ample time for explanation and counselling from all the professionals, including experienced social workers. Where necessary the person and carers should be guided into the various support networks that exist to help any given problem. The memory clinic should act as the centre of a network, where referrals for help and advice come in, and also go out to other agencies perhaps better suited to a particular problem. The memory clinic will also have a research and educational role, developing a pool of people who may be suitable for specialised research projects, medical, psychiatric and social. The clinic should run courses on management, treatment, etc., and hence disseminate the expertise it develops. Health authority and social services should see it as the resource centre for all aspects of care of the elderly mentally infirm.

How a memory clinic works

To show how a memory clinic works on a practical level (and in case someone you know is referred to one so that you know what to expect), I have set out below how a typical memory clinic would work and the procedures involved.

- Referrals should be comprehensively discussed with regards to suitability for the memory clinic or day hospital. When necessary a domiciliary visit should be carried out.
- Appointments will be dealt with and transport will be arranged if necessary.
- Where necessary notes should be requested from other agencies, i.e. hospitals, social services, GPs and community psychiatric nurses. If there is very little information about the patient, then check with the geriatric office in case any more details are forthcoming.
- Prior to attendance at the memory clinic, all the notes for the clients coming to the clinic will be checked, as will those for review.
- Appointment:
  9.00 am clients arrive.
  9.15 am will be seen by the doctors and the rest of the team.
  1.00 pm team meet to discuss client and formulate plan.
- Plan is then explained to client and relatives. Immediately afterwards the team will meet to discuss the review cases and appoint a key worker who will ensure that all services have been arranged. They will also telephone or contact the client or relatives two months after the review to check that services have happened and that no new problems have arisen and report back to the team.
- After the clinic a record will be kept on the clients who have attended and those who have been reviewed.
- The doctor will write to all the services involved on behalf of the team.
- During the memory clinic the roles are:
  Nurses will fill in as many details of history (family and medical) as possible. They will give the health education booklet out and discuss with client and carers any worries they

may have, explaining conditions if necessary.

Doctors will do the mini-mental assessment (see box), full physical and blood tests and talk to the relatives.

Social worker will talk to relatives regarding social aspects and explain about the relatives' support group.

Occupational therapist assesses client's ADL (activities of daily living).

- Computer memory testing will be done by a member of the team. Domiciliary visits will be done by one or two members of the team, either before or after the memory clinic visit.

MINI-MENTAL STATE QUESTIONNAIRE

This is a detailed assessment of orientation, attention, calculation and language, the person being scored out of a maximum of 30. However it is not only the score that is important but how the person managed the test, their motivation, etc. A skilled assessor can gain a lot more information than simply the final score.

Orientation

Maximum score	Actual score	Question
5		What is the (year), (season), (date), (day), and (month)?
5		Where are we – (country), (city), (suburb), (street), (hospital)?
3		Name three objects, one second to say each. Then repeat them until he/she learns all three if possible. Count trials and record. Trials = Number =

Attention and calculation

5

Spell WORLD forwards and backwards or do serial 7s (take seven from 100 repeatedly). 1 point for each correct.

3

As for the three objects repeated above (1 point for each correct).

Language

2

Name two objects, e.g. pen and watch.

1

Repeat the following: 'No ifs, ands or buts'.

3

Follow a three-stage command: 'Take a paper in your right hand, fold it in half, and put it on the floor'.

3

Read and obey the following: 'Close your eyes' (1 point). 'Write a sentence' (1 point). 'Copy this design' (1 point).

8

Legal aspects

If a parent worn out by unemployment, debt or marital trauma feels that they are about to abuse their child, a cry for help will unleash a planned response from numerous caring agencies, a response insisted upon by law. This can ultimately involve the abused or the abuser being removed from the family home. Contrast this to the exhausted carer who makes a similar plea for help before they abuse their elderly demented relative, and one finds that no compulsory help is forthcoming, the law is not automatically involved. It has long been recognised that a minimum legal framework imposing compulsory duties on statutory bodies and perhaps individuals is long overdue. The Law Commission recognised this and incorporated a similar requirement into its 1993 report on mentally incapacitated and other vulnerable adults – Public Law Protection (HMSO).

The majority of the elderly mentally frail live in the community (only about 6 per cent live in institutions) and they and their carers, given the right amount of help, would like them to remain there. Surely the approach of a caring society will be to keep as many people out of institutions as possible, and those that need either medical or social 'homes' should then have a right of entry for their own safety and well being. Any legislation, however, must be seen to enhance the independence of the individual and not be seen as a way to reduce individual liberty. The admission to a rest home should be a positive choice for the elderly person, and if the issue

We have in mind the donor who is no longer fully capable when he grants the Enduring Power of Attorney, even though he still has sufficient capacity to create the power. This is likely to be a very common case in practice where (as will be most usual) the donor is elderly.

Agency

A nominated person (the agent) acts on a frail person's behalf within specified instructions. This is especially seen in the social security system, where a pensioner will nominate someone to collect their benefits from the post office. The agent can only collect the money, and they must then hand it to the person concerned. Many people use this form of help to enable friends, neighbours or home helps to collect pensions.

There is a set procedure for this form of transaction. The pensioner deletes 'I acknowledge receipt of the above sum' which is printed on the pension. They then sign it as usual, and write and sign on the back 'I am unable to go to the Post Office and I authorise (signature)'. This must be witnessed by someone other than the agent. The agent also has to sign the following: 'I am today the authorised agent. I certify that the payee is alive today. I acknowledge receipt of the amount shown overleaf which I will pay to the payee forthwith' (signature).

Disabled Persons Act 1986

This Act was passed by Parliament in 1986, but its 18 sections are being brought into force gradually. The Act gives disabled people four rights:

- The right to representation – in cases of mental or severe physical incapacity the local authority can appoint a representative on behalf of the disabled person or ask a voluntary organisation to appoint someone.
- The right to assessment – this includes any disabled person who asks for services from the local authority under section 2 of the

Chronically Sick and Disabled Persons Act 1970.

• The right to information – if a disabled person receives a service from social services then they must also be informed of the other services available and any other relevant services provided by other local authorities.

• The right to consultation – the Chronically Sick and Disabled Persons Act 1970 states that certain councils and committees should have a disabled person or someone with special knowledge on that committee. The 1986 Act states that the person can only be appointed after consultation with organisations of disabled people.

The living will

There are many people who fear becoming old and 'senile' because once they become mentally frail they will no longer be able to tell people what their wishes are, especially in relation to medical treatment. Currently the position is that doctors dealing with the mentally frail are governed by what is known as 'good medical practice': because the person concerned cannot give consent, measures are taken 'in their best interests'. Most teams of professionals dealing with the elderly in the UK would discuss the dilemma with the person's family, although the latter have no legal force to sway the doctors one way or the other (enduring powers of attorney specifically exclude medical matters). 'Good medical practice' may mean that a person undergoes an operation or is given some form of treatment that his family and friends know would have been refused had the person been competent.

In the United States there has been legislation in many states to try to insist on the autonomy of the person under consideration being paramount, and to do this the person must make a statement basically saying how far he would like doctors to go in the event of him/her becoming incapable of giving informed consent. Obviously such a statement must be made before any brain damage has occurred. This statement is called a living will and describes a form of anticipated consent. The following is an example of a living will:

It is my express wish that if I develop an acute or chronic

cerebral illness which results in a substantial loss of dignity, and the opinions of two independent physicians indicate that my condition is unlikely to be reversible, any separate illness which may threaten my life should not be given active treatment.

In the USA this is a legally binding document, but this is not the case in the UK. The above example is only one type of document that could be drawn up; some people would perhaps want to refuse life-support machines or mutilating operations but would want antibiotics or other 'invasive' medical treatments. The UK is certainly different in its treatment of the very mentally frail and few doctors here would deem it appropriate to put someone with advanced dementia onto life-support machines or subject them to major operations without much thought and significant benefit to the individual. Good medical practice, however, still leaves important decisions in the hands of comparative strangers whose moral and ethical values may differ markedly from the person they are treating.

That is not to say that good practice does not currently allow for the extremely mentally frail with other severe illness to die pain free and with dignity. The British Medical Association (BMA) was initially reluctant to acknowledge the need for living wills, and in the 1980s its Ethics Committee reported they were quasi-legal documents that could arouse fear in some people. The debate has continued, however, and new impetus has been given to the topic by the large numbers of people affected by AIDS. The Terrence Higgins Trust, a leading AIDS charity, has produced its own living will and distributes copies free of charge. Because HIV-related diseases and AIDS affects a predominantly younger population than dementia, it has focused attention away from age and onto the point at issue, personal autonomy. The latest statements from the BMA encourage acceptance of the principle and debate on the issue. It is a topic arousing Parliamentary interest with a view to giving it some legal status as is the case abroad.

The need for discussion around this very important topic is evident. I feel very strongly that many people would contemplate writing a living will because currently many institutions caring for the elderly mentally frail are so under-funded and under-staffed that the reality of life in these places fills many people with dread.

In such circumstances, however, a living will coming into effect must never be used to decrease the funding to this vital part of the health service merely because of a cynical anticipated lack of demand later. The living will debate is only valid if more resources are placed into this sector so that the reality for the elderly mentally infirm in care is of excellent architecture with enviable surroundings, single rooms with bath and toilet, and sufficient care staff properly trained to ensure life with dignity. A living will for intercurrent illness would then truly enhance a person's autonomy.

Abuse of elderly people

In the late 1970s articles concerning the physical abuse of old people began appearing in medical journals and the lay press. There was a flurry of debate and then interest waned. Even though reports appeared at regular intervals documenting isolated cases and occasionally large-scale institutional abuse, it was the physical and sexual abuse of children that caught the public imagination and has retained a firm hold on it. Recent scandals of systematic cruelty and abuse in old people's homes only hold the headlines for a few days, whereas the Cleveland affair has rarely left the media since its occurrence. The recognition of abuse of old people is probably at the same stage as that of child abuse in the 1970s – the explosion has yet to come.

What is old age abuse? The definitions are varied and range from the broad idea of misuse of power to the more hardened physical or sexual assault. In between are the concepts of emotional, psychological and verbal abuse. What we do know is that there is very little research in this field compared to that on child abuse. Many consider it a moral problem, a concern of society, a reflection of its attitudes and concepts of what is acceptable. We know it exists but there is much debate as to the sheer size of the problem. Some social workers are beginning to take the problem very seriously and their preliminary studies indicate that up to 5 per cent of their social work cases involve some aspect of abuse to an old person.

There are eight areas of abuse:

• Assault, including forced feeding

- Deprivation of nutrition/neglect
- Drugs – deprivation and overdosing
- Emotional/verbal, including intimidation
- Sexual
- Deprivation of help and aids when disabled
- Involuntary isolation
- Financial

My first thoughts on this problem are that most carers perform their caring duties as best they can, and that a close relationship between any two people will have its good and bad times. For most even the bad times will involve nothing more than raised voices and harsh words spoken. A small minority of old people will have carers who are emotionally unstable, with violent tendencies to match; they are at great risk but are hopefully identifiable, as the carer will be known about. The unknown quantity of other cases will involve carers who have been put under intolerable stress by their caring burden; something happens, they snap and the person is abused. It can never be condoned but it can be understood. And who is the more guilty, the carer who finally caves in or the rest of us for allowing things to reach such an awful position?

Some work has been done on trying to identify the elderly and their carers most at risk from abuse. It seems that most carers who later abuse have been to their GP before the event. They go with minor ailments, but if recognised and asked they talk of the increasing burden of caring and of some resentment creeping into the relationship with the sufferer. Indeed what they are trying to say, but dare not, is that they fear abusing the other person. There then usually occurs a triggering factor or 'last straw', such as a bout of incontinence or disturbed sleep, and the abuse occurs. A chilling comment by an abuser was 'It's much easier after the first time'. A large group of carers agreed to be interviewed in a recent research study. Two-thirds of the group admitted losing their tempers with the relative and one-fifth said that they occasionally resorted to shaking or hitting the person. A fifth also reported that the sufferers tried to hit them, especially those that were confused, and it was this confused group that were most likely to be hit themselves. The most comprehensive (and only large scale) survey of elder abuse was carried out by Ogg and Bennett in 1992. They found that on a random sample of elderly people 5 per cent had been verbally abused and 2 per cent physically or financially abused. A survey of people in a caring role showed that 10 per cent admitted verbally abusing an elderly person and 1 per cent said they had physically abused them. If reproduced nationally these figures would equate to over one million elderly people being verbally abused and half a million physically abused.

There was a stereotyped picture of the sort of elderly person most likely to be abused (in any setting). Most at risk were thought to be very elderly females, chronically confused, unable to converse normally, tending to have no purposeful activity between meals. The person had negative personality traits such as incontinence, unpleasant behaviour (biting, spitting, masturbating), dysphasia (difficulty speaking) and disturbed sleep patterns.

This stereotype may match many victims but as more research is carried out into this problem, both here and in the US, what is revealed is the diversity of the condition and not its sameness. Some US studies show that it is spouse abuse (usually male to female) continued into old age that is the most common. In other studies nearly as many men as women were being abused. There were no stereotypes in terms of class, race, etc. It would seem that any elderly person may be at risk of abuse. In the US Holly Ramsey-Klawsnik has made a personal study of sexual abuse of elderly people. In this condition women victims do outnumber men, but males are abused. She points out that the most at risk are those in powerless positions (either physical or mental frailty) and that the abusers are overwhelmingly men.

In the UK, less thought has been given to the theories concerning abuse of older people. The carer stress theory has gained most support and as most carers are women they have been identified and labelled using this approach. A typically stressed carer will feel lonely and isolated; probably they will have confessed to someone (perhaps a GP) the desire to stop caring, saying that the elderly person is most awkward when they are most tired. The resentment is initially only shown in private but as the stress and burn-out continues this changes. The help the carer gives becomes more harsh, an arm up becomes a pull, then a jerk and finally a shove onto the floor. Physical restraints may be used (tying into a chair or bed) and there may be excessive use of medication to keep a person quiet and give the carer some rest.

Research work in the US, however, questions this theory as the main one, its findings showing that the psychological state of the carer was the most important predictive feature of abusive episodes. This work, substantiated by others, did not try to imply a lessening of the stress of a caring role but indicated that as most carers feel like abusing but don't, then the actual serious abusers could be looked at more closely. It found that they suffered from major psychological or psychiatric disturbance including alcoholism, drug dependency and disturbed mental states. Placing them in a caring role over someone physically or mentally frail was beyond their capabilities and abuse was the result. Much more work is needed in this area in the UK before this complex question can be better answered.

Carers themselves may be able to indicate and verbalise that all is not well; knowing the home situation, health care professionals should then be able to recognise these elements of stress and gently and sympathetically explore the issue. The sufferer, especially if confused, may not be able to tell anyone, and for many elderly people the fear of them being 'put away' or their carer removed, essentially leading to the same thing happening, means that they keep quiet and suffer. Physical symptoms and signs may indicate that something is wrong. An elderly person cowering and obviously frightened of being touched is suspicious. Thumb-print bruising and bruising in odd places such as the front of the chest, in the hair-line and around the jaw and eye could indicate abuse. Bruises of different ages and signs of general neglect are also worrying. There are no absolute signs: often it is a pattern of features over a period of time that lead to the diagnosis being considered.

Elderly people can bruise easily, (transparent skin syndrome or photoageing). Diagnosis of physical abuse should only be made after exhaustive enquiries, questioning victims and possible perpetrators in a non-threatening way. Guidelines are necessary and help both health and social services. Tower Hamlets, a pioneer in this field, have adopted the use of the term 'inadequate care' to help in this process. Because the diagnosis of abuse may be extremely difficult and threatening to all concerned, it may be better to use the term inadequate care as pioneered in the US.

Professionals especially are happier to investigate a case of inadequate care – defined thus: the presence of unmet needs for the elderly person – than a case of elder abuse. On a practical and pragmatic level abuse may never be definitely diagnosed, but this does not stop professionals from assessing a situation and helping in many ways. If abuse is found it can be dealt with as necessary.

Obviously abuse is not confined to relatives and other carers at home. It occurs in institutions (old people's homes and hospitals) ranging from the institutional abuse of a lack of privacy to perform the most basic of tasks, to actual physical abuse in these places. This information comes from major enquiries, Coroners' inquests, consumer response, Registered Home Act tribunals, Social Service Inspectorate and the media. In old people's homes the staff have low status and pay and in many cases very low morale. Some have no training at all. Long-stay hospital wards can sometimes fare little better.

Solutions

What can we do about this growing area of concern? Carers were asked what their requirements were, using this as a starting point. They not unreasonably wanted assessments at regular intervals of their dependent sufferer. New problems could then be referred to the correct agency and appropriate back-up provided. Medical treatment was seen as very important, especially of the intercurrent problems that many frail handicapped elderly people develop, e.g. constipation, incontinence, hearing and sight problems, as well as dental disorders and foot trouble. Information, advice and counselling on the major underlying medical problem was seen as vital, be it Alzheimer's, Parkinson's or whatever. Practical help was necessary as well as regular breaks. It was interesting to note, however, that breaks did not bring down the stress levels by very much; this was only achieved by long-term residential care. Financial support was also necessary. Residential care was seen as needed and necessary by many carers.

Institutions need a different set of solutions. One area of change is in the designing of patterns of care, and not their imposition. Much, however, is dependent on resource allocation. The provision of small units with single rooms and bathrooms, adequate numbers of care assistants – paid well and trained for the job – allowing choice and privacy, does not come cheaply.

Interest in the problem of abuse of elderly people is undergoing a marked resurgence of interest. A new charity – Action on Elder Abuse – has been formed with the mission statement: to prevent abuse in old age by promoting changes in policy and practice through raising awareness, education, promoting research and providing information. This organisation is initially aimed at educating and informing professionals working in the field as to the importance of the topic and where to go for research information. Hopefully it will develop further into a major pressure group, aimed at establishing interest at local and central government level. Elder abuse is not yet identified as a social problem. To achieve this status it must be recognised as a problem by society which in turn puts pressure on government to achieve change. Society is becoming increasingly better informed about the topic and as professionals become aware more and more cases are being discovered.

Guidelines have been mentioned previously. They are in place in only a minority of health authorities but in an increasing number of local authorities. The major obstacle to full scale reform is the lack of legislation. Hopefully this too will change as elder abuse becomes a bona fide social problem on a par with child abuse and other forms of family violence. Currently most authorities use the case conference format for dissemination and discussion of information. A multidisciplinary group of people (social worker, GP, district nurse, hospital doctor, home help organiser, etc.) try to resolve the issues to the best of their ability. Some cases may need the involvement of the police but legal or other specialist help may also be needed. The client should be present (for at least part of the proceedings) as well as the alleged abuser (this obviously has to be handled sensitively). Many groups such as Action on Elder Abuse and Age Concern are putting this issue on the political and media agenda. They feel, quite rightly, that the interests of the elderly person are paramount. The vulnerable old person in the community currently has no rights to ensure that they are protected against abuse in its widest sense. The alarming paradox that there is a legal duty to protect children from abuse but that there is no such legal duty to protect equally vulnerable adults has to be laid at the politicians' door.

The law needs to be changed so that this particularly vulnerable group is protected and their human rights upheld. Age Concern feel that this may involve a Charter of Rights which is legally binding and could extend to institutions; that there should be a proper complaints procedure such as an ombudsman, guardian or advocate system and that this concept of advocacy would allow the frail person's views to be expressed. The problem is complex but there is now no doubt that it is here to stay and we should act now.

Action on Elder Abuse
Astral House
1268 London Road
London SW16 4ER
Tel 0181 679 2648
Fax 0181 679 6069

For further reading:
Elder abuse: concepts, theories and interventions, Bennett, G and Kingston, P, Chapman and Hall, 1993

9

Areas of conflict

In this chapter the potential areas of conflict between sufferer, carer and the medical professionals will be discussed. I have concentrated on two main areas:

- Obtaining medical help
- Discharge from hospital

Obtaining medical help

This may not seem a problem area at first glance, but so many families have complained to me about it that I have included it.

For most of us our main medical carer is the general practitioner. If the medical problem is serious then the GP should see the person at home, especially if the patient is old and somewhat frail. Obtaining this visit should not be difficult and if the person concerned or the carer feels that they cannot get to the surgery, then a GP should visit. In all other instances, unless the GP routinely sees his/her elderly patients at home, one should try and get to the surgery. Many people complain that they cannot get past the receptionist for either a home visit or a chance to speak to the doctor. The receptionist has a job to do and most manage to find out the problem, fit in appointments, do a host of other things and remain friendly. If however you feel you must speak to the doctor then insist on doing so. Most receptionists only protect the doctor so far, and are then under orders to pass the problem on.

Any difficulties with medication should be reported at once so that it can be stopped if the GP thinks it advisable. Anyone on repeat prescriptions should see their doctor regularly and have the need for the medicine reassessed. Most elderly people can stop taking their medication safely once the acute problem is over; few should be on drugs long term, and then only under supervision. If a hospital appointment changes the medication, be sure to let the GP know. The hospital should automatically let the GP know anyway, but it sometimes takes many weeks for letters to arrive.

Many elderly people and their carers worry about health issues but often keep the worries to themselves. The GP should be told of any concerns so that the person can be listened to, examined and then either reassured or the problem dealt with. No symptom should be taken as a sign of old age, especially if the problem involves confusional episodes, falls, incontinence or decreased mobility. The GP can perform many of the screening tests necessary to rule out treatable causes, but may then want to refer the person to a specialist. There is now an ideal opportunity to regularly have some of these issues discussed. GPs are now obliged to offer a screening/assessment visit to all elderly people over the age of 75. The GP may perform the visit (or invite you to the surgery) or they may delegate the screening to a practice nurse. The areas that have to be asked about are sight, hearing, feet, diet, weight and blood pressure but an elderly person can add any issue that is worrying them. This can prove to be an excellent time to get all one's questions answered.

Many carers feel that their relative was not referred to a specialist soon enough. This dilemma is often a difficult one for in some cases the specialist cannot offer any more help than is already being given. However in most difficult cases a 'second opinion' is no bad thing and at least it can reassure sufferer and carers that no stone is being left unturned to help. Most GPs will not refuse a referral to another doctor unless they really feel that it is not justified.

Hopefully real areas of conflict between patient/carer and doctor will be few, but as a last resort one is entitled to leave one GP's books and join another. Help is available from the Family Health Services Agency (FHSA) – (the GP's watchdog) or Citizens Advice

Bureaux. GP's are not only the gatekeepers to further medical tests and advice; they also can hold sway over the local district nurses and health visitors. Changes in these services often have to go through the GP, but it is worth contacting them directly if there are any problems. The fact that a GP practice is a fund-holder should not affect the care given in any way. Should a problem arise that is apparently linked to finance, it is best first to discuss it openly with the GP. If you are still not satisfied then go to the FHSA or local Citizen's Advice Bureau.

Some carers report a reluctance on the part of GPs to deal with the acute conditions that can occur in someone with dementia. These acute-on-chronic crises can be very frightening and yet the problem is seen in the light of the underlying dementia, i.e. the person has one 'untreatable' condition which leads to the assumption that all other things occurring are untreatable. Nothing could be more wrong – acute illnesses resolve in the confused elderly as in other people. What is wrong is to allow an already confused person to become even more disorientated and upset through ignorance. In difficult cases it is often possible to ask the GP to arrange for a home visit by a specialist (geriatrician or psychogeriatrician). This allows for a thorough airing of views and anxieties, lets the specialist see the sufferer in their own home, lets them meet the carer and listen to them and hopefully also allows the specialist to meet the GP at the patient's home and discuss the case.

Respite breaks and holiday breaks are initially arranged through the GP, who then contacts the relevant organisation. Obviously as much notice as possible should be given. Admission to hospital for whatever reason is usually based on the decision of the GP. Some elderly people are extremely reluctant to consider hospitalisation and need great reassurance; the GP will know of any other schemes that may be available to keep an elderly person at home and yet give them the care they need. Some areas have 'hospital at home' schemes, with intensive nursing hours provided; on other occasions the local day hospital may be appropriate. Problems do arise when either the person themself or a carer feels that they should be in hospital but the GP disagrees. This can usually be talked through and a solution agreeable to both parties arrived at, but should there be any medical change in the person's condition then the GP should be called back.

Good GPs are worth their weight in gold; bad ones can mean misery to a frail old person and their carers. Their gatekeeping role is a very powerful one indeed.

Discharge from hospital

This particular area can be fraught with problems and has come to the government's attention. There are now very strict guidelines given to hospitals concerning the discharge process and these guidelines must be followed. The ideal should be as follows.

The medical problem is over, the person treated and looking forward to returning home. Any carers involved are happy and have met with the hospital staff concerning the discharge. Mobility problems have been identified and a home visit has been carried out by the hospital therapy staff. Prior to discharge the multi-disciplinary team meet and all contribute their views. A care plan is agreed with the patient and family and is written up by the social worker. If this requires a lot of new services, the community care manager either automatically agrees it or calls a case conference. A discharge date is set and each member carries out any special tasks (social worker will order services after talking with patient and carer, the ward staff order the ambulance, the junior doctor will write a discharge note and organise any medication to go with the patient). Patient and carer are kept informed of all actions as is the GP and the discharge goes ahead uneventfully. The key is communication.

Unfortunately many discharges do not resemble the above at all. Many excuses are given but inevitably the failure is in communication. There are no easy answers but wards and professionals alike should not get away with bad practice. If the discharge procedure goes wrong then the people concerned should know about it. Vigorous complaints are one way to change and hopefully improve the service. No one likes to complain but without such guided criticism mistakes will continue to occur. Complaining itself is no easy process but again this has been recognised by government and each hospital has a complaints procedure which should go into action immediately, offering a reply within 14 days. To ensure that the problem gets looked into the complaint must be in writing and preferably addressed to the service manager and/or the hospital's public relations officer. In very serious cases a copy of the letter should also go to the hospital's Chief Executive (the trust's boss). This is not to say that many difficulties cannot be resolved by speaking to the various people concerned but a change of practice needs a letter.

A special difficulty occurs when a carer feels that a person cannot return home. This happens extremely frequently, and I have seen a vast increase in this particular problem since the NHS and community have been so starved of resources. What seems to happen is that the admission to hospital because of an acute illness provides the break needed in which a total evaluation can occur of the difficulties at home as suffered by the patient and carer. There is always a long history of increasing failure to cope at home, with either no other help sought or that help having failed in some way. It is at its most desperate when dealing with the elderly mentally confused, where the resources are indeed limited. Bear in mind that carers have to be pretty desperate to say 'No' to the massed authority of the hospital hierarchy.

If a carer feels concerned about the impending discharge of a relative, then they must speak out as soon as possible. In many cases discussion with the various team members involved will allow for a compromise, in that more help is provided if possible. If this does not allay fears sufficiently, the carer and other people involved should meet up with the consultant concerned; it may be appropriate to invite others to this meeting, such as the social worker dealing with the case, etc. In cases of real conflict then a case conference should be held, involving the multidisciplinary team as well as the carers, community agencies involved and the person concerned. Carers should ask for such a meeting if they are really unhappy about an impending discharge; it allows for everyone to say their piece and for the carer especially to point out the realities of life to the other conference members. The point of the conference is to arrive at a solution acceptable to everyone.

Where the patient is able to communicate well, their wishes are paramount, and if they want to return home then as much as possible will be done to ensure this. Often this involves the taking of considerable risks, and carers are sometimes counselled to accept this. Where the patient is mentally frail, however, and not able to vocalise their wishes clearly, the task is harder. The choice is usually between the patient going home against the carer's wishes and entering some form of institution. These decisions are never easy and there are pressures on both sides. On the consultant's mind is his/her commitment to other people who need the beds and services of the hospital, as well as the multidisciplinary team's appraisal of whether or not a return home is feasible. The carers on the other hand have often been through it all before. Their concern for a relative may be so great, however, as to cloud their judgment and not allow them to see alternatives. There are no easy answers. The two sides must trust each other and in most cases a reasonably amicable solution is found. The equation at the moment is far too heavily weighted in favour of the hospital; the needs of consumer and carer have to be more forcibly stated and, more importantly, acted upon.

Research and the future

Drugs Therapy

In the last few years exciting new research has been reported in both the medical and the lay press. There has been a surge of optimism akin to the breakthrough use of L-dopa in the treatment of Parkinson's disease. Is this optimism warranted? Or are we raising false hopes, too soon?

It is well known that the most damaging chemical loss in Alzheimer's disease is in the chemical acetylcholine (ACh). A lot of work has therefore gone into testing a group of drugs – the anticholinesterases – which stop the breakdown of ACh. The drug described most widely is 9-amino – 1, 2, 3, 4 tetrahydroacridine, (THA or Tacrine*). Studies have shown evidence of a small but significant reduction in the rate of decline in mental state and some improvements in cover assessments of the patients. Not all people were helped however, and of the sample of patients tested in the trials only 30% to 50% showed any sign of improvement, which is an inconclusive result, and the benefits were small. There is thus space for a little optimism but drug treatment as a major advance is still in the research stage.

The social research is moving away from examining the patient and towards understanding the position of the carers and putting their viewpoint across. This is vitally important; for too long this group of people has been taken for granted and their needs ignored. More work is also being done teaching the professionals who come into contact with the elderly and especially the elderly mentally confused. Dramatic changes in policy, finance, resources, etc., will only take place if those in the position to influence such things are aware of the problem. Much research work has shown that, from medical students to politicians, there is a lack of knowledge and interest in the problems of the elderly. This will only change with education and the elderly themselves becoming more of a pressure group to press for reform.

Possible causes

In the field of dementia many exciting developments have exploded on to the scene concerning both the cause and possible prevention of Alzheimer's disease. The top three current theories can be listed:

- Genetic
- Aluminium
- Viral

The first two especially, and perhaps all three, may be interrelated and a brief discussion of them all will explain where scientific minds are leading, with the hope of dramatic announcements in the next few years.

Genetic

There have always been some cases of Alzheimer's disease that have appeared to run in families. The most well researched ones have been found where the condition has occurred in younger people (like the original cases Alzheimer described). We know however that this type of dementia in younger people is very rare (0.1 per cent of total cases of dementia). There are in fact only 12 families world wide currently being studied with this rare and obviously directly inherited form of the disease. In studying these families it did seem that the condition was passed on to the next generation but not in a very straightforward pattern – one could not predict which offspring if any would develop dementia. We now know that Alzheimer's disease becomes much more common as we get older (as high as 20 per cent of the over-80 age group are affected). Being quite common, it then becomes hard to know if the dementia is passed on in a family or whether or not the dementia has occurred in the next generation by chance; one has to wait for the children to grow old, and they have a 20 per cent chance of developing dementia anyway.

Someone then noticed that all cases of Down's syndrome developed a condition identical to Alzheimer's disease before they died young. It had been recognised for a long time that people suffering from Down's syndrome 'aged' very quickly, but it was not until this observation about their dementia was made that its importance was realised. Studies on the brains of people dying with Down's syndrome show all the changes seen in those dying with Alzheimer's disease. Now, we don't know what causes Alzheimer's disease but we do know the cause of Down's syndrome; in the majority of cases it is due to a fault in the chromosomes, the tiny bits of genetic material that are found in each cell and that originally come from each parent.

Each of us has 23 pairs of chromosomes, 46 chromosomes in all, in

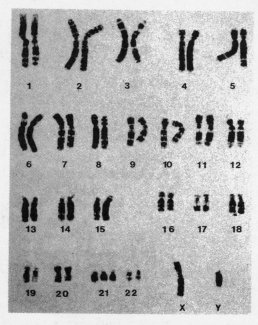

Karyotype showing the arrangement of chromosomes in a male with Down's syndrome (trisomy–21).

each cell. The only exceptions are sperm cells in men and ova (the egg cells) in women – they have 23 single chromosomes, half the usual number. When a baby is conceived by the fusion of a sperm and an ovum, the full complement of 23 pairs of chromosomes is achieved, the baby's cells containing a mixture of the mother's and father's chromosomes. In a Down's syndrome baby something goes wrong with this process and chromosome pair number 21 ends up with an extra bit of genetic material. This tiny excess produces all the abnormalities associated with the condition, including the development of changes exactly like Alzheimer's disease. Each chromosome is made up of hundreds of genes (small sequences of genetic information controlling a bit of the workings of the body). It seems likely therefore that as chromosome 21 has the gene that produces Alzheimer's disease in Down's syndrome, the same chromosome should have a gene for Alzheimer's disease in non-Down's-syndrome people with, or who will develop, Alzheimer's disease.

The topic is made more complicated by the finding that chromosome 21 may not be the only genetic source of the problem. Researchers have found families with early onset dementia where chromosome 14 is abnormal and some where chromosome 19 is probably at fault. Many researchers now feel that these genetic changes are more important than the original lead with chromosome 21 and Down's syndrome, which may have given the impetus but will not be the answer. In addition medical interest is now focusing upon the role of a protein in the body called amyloid – more specifically beta-amyloid. The amyloid is governed by the amyloid APP gene and this abnormality also appears to run in families, making it another familial form. It appears that some cases of dementia are caused by a gene for the precursor stage of beta-amyloid being in the wrong place causing this protein to be abnormally deposited all over the brain. What is unknown is the relative significance of these findings and how important to the general population are the findings of an abnormal chromosome 21, chromosome 14 and the misplaced gene for beta-amyloid (and even if the beta-amyloid gene is related to the other chromosomal abnormalities and in what way).

Finding a gene on a chromosome may sound easy but in fact it is extremely difficult. Researchers in both the UK and the USA are currently working on this project and they expect to be able to identify the gene soon. This will then open up many more research possibilities. Once identified it can be looked for in people currently suffering from Alzheimer's disease. Is it present in every case? If not, do those who appear to have Alzheimer's disease but who do not have the gene really have Alzheimer's disease, and not some other similar condition? Is the gene passed from generation to generation? If present in normal healthy people, will they go on to develop the disease? As you can see it is exciting research but it throws up many difficult questions. Should you look for and tell someone they are carrying a gene that may mean that they develop dementia, a condition for which there is currently no cure?

Most of the experts working in this field think it is unlikely that carrying the gene alone will automatically mean that the person will develop dementia, unless they are in one of those families where the disease presents very early. It is felt that the gene being present means that you are more at risk than someone without the gene, but that you still need a trigger to set the whole thing off. More and more attention is being paid to environmental triggers – abnormalities in the environment which can act as general hazards – the theory being that such triggers, when put together with a genetically predisposed individual, result in dementia developing.

Aluminium

A breakthrough came with the ability to use electron microscopes and other sophisticated techniques to study the brains of people who had died of Alzheimer's disease. At the centre of the damaged brain tissue and tangled brain cells there appeared to be something – a minute piece of aluminium (alumino-silicate).

This discovery was extremely exciting. However, did the aluminium cause the neurological changes or did the changes come first and the aluminium get there merely as a waste product? The question is still not answered. We know that aluminium is the commonest metal in the earth's crust. It is thus part of our water supply and is taken up by the plants that we eat. It has always been thought that our bodies only take up a limited amount of aluminium and that we excrete the majority of it (we do not need it to any great extent). Some years ago, however, when renal dialysis was starting, it was noted that some people during their treatment were getting progressively confused and looked like they were developing a dementia. This was thoroughly investigated and it was found that the dialysis fluid used to treat the patients contained a high level of aluminium and it was this that was causing the people to appear demented. As soon as this was realised the aluminium in the dialysis fluid was removed and the problem disappeared. Thus we do know that aluminium can be harmful to the brain in certain circumstances.

There are some parts of the world where the concentrations of aluminium in the soil and water are extremely high. Studies in these areas have revealed some fascinating facts. Most studies have been done in small communities and islands in the western Pacific, where not only is the concentration of aluminium very high but there are high rates of neurological diseases such as Alzheimer's disease and Parkinson's disease. Are the two facts causally related? At the moment no one is certain, but very recently it was reported in the press that some areas in Britain have water supplies that contain high levels of aluminium, and these same areas have high rates of Alzheimer's disease. The response of the water boards was predictable – there was absolutely no danger from these levels of aluminium. However all agreed to ensure that the levels would be reduced in the near future. Questions are now being asked about the safety of using aluminium cooking pots and pans. At a recent conference I attended an 'expert' was asked this question. He replied that there was no proof whatsoever that aluminium pans were in any way harmful – but he'd thrown his out.

The role of aluminium remains unanswered. It seems unlikely that it will prove to be the cause in its own right. More likely is that it may be one of the triggers that set the neurological abnormalities off in a genetically predisposed individual.

Viral

Viruses are tiny particles that invade the body and cause diseases ranging from the common cold to hepatitis (inflammation of the liver) and AIDS. Depending on the type they can enter the body easily (in the air in the case of influenza) or only with difficulty (in body fluids such as blood and semen in the case of AIDS). Viruses themselves vary in shape and size and in the ease with which they can be isolated and seen.

There are many disease processes of which we are unsure as to the cause, and many scientists feel that these conditions may be caused by viruses that have yet to be isolated; for example, some doctors believe that rheumatoid arthritis and multiple sclerosis are such conditions. The story with MS is very interesting. It is much more common in temperate climates and in certain countries, e.g. UK, Eire and New Zealand. There is also an unequal distribution within a country, the disease being concentrated in the more remote country areas. It was then noted that these were the most heavily used areas for sheep rearing and that there is a disease of sheep called scrapie that has some of the features of multiple sclerosis. Scrapie is known to be caused by a virus. However, despite much hunting, no virus has been found in MS.

Viruses can produce new disease symptoms many years after the original infectious disease. For example, the measles virus can get into the nervous tissue, where it lies dormant; many years later, though, it can cause a disease called sclerosing panencephalitis, a low-grade inflammation of the brain. This delayed effect is due to what is called a slow virus.

It is also known that viruses can cause dementia the so-called Prion Dementias. An extremely rare condition called Jakob Creutzfeldt disease has been shown to be caused by a virus. This virus can be passed on to other people, despite the fact that it remains within the nervous system of those affected, i.e. it shouldn't be infectious. Its potential for transmission was noted when the condition was found to have been passed on within a group of cannibals; presumably eating the brain of an infected person was enough to transmit the virus. Modern reports have shown that the virus has been passed on by accidental inoculation – doctors and technicians dealing with cerebrospinal fluid and nervous tissue samples are at special risk. There is ongoing medical debate which has now become an issue in the political arena, as to whether BSE (Bovine Spongiform Encephalopathy) 'Mad Cow Disease', a viral dementia of animals can ever be passed to humans in the food chain. The AIDS virus is the latest to be shown to cause dementia, albeit in a small proportion of sufferers.

Treatment

We have seen the first tissue implants into the brains of sufferers of

Parkinson's disease. The tissue has either been from their own adrenal glands (situated on top of the kidneys) or from aborted foetuses, and contains the cells capable of producing the neurochemical transmitter dopamine (the substance deficient in the disease). The tissue is placed via a thin needle into the brain, with the hope that the cells will 'take' and produce dopamine.

Many carers have asked whether or not the same sort of operation will soon be available for sufferers of Alzheimer's disease. The answer is almost definitely not. Unlike Parkinson's disease, the deficits in Alzheimer's disease are multiple and very complex and accompanied by structural changes in the nerve cells. The door cannot be slammed shut, however; tissue brain transplants have a science fiction, fantasy aura about them, but in the case of Parkinson's disease they have become a reality. As research continues, possibilities concerning prevention, treatment and cure of Alzheimer's disease may well become realities.

New types of dementia are being discovered almost daily. The latest ones include Prion disease, Cortico-Basal Degeneration and Cortical Lewy Body disease. Some of them are extremely complex microscopic-based changes and their true place in the overall picture is unclear. What is clear, however, is that Alzheimer's disease may soon have to be called Alzheimer's diseases. It is beginning to appear that what was once thought to be a single disease is now made up of many sub-types. As the technology advances, we may soon be talking about the various ways in which these sub-types can be treated or even prevented by drugs. As the role of genetics gets bigger and bigger there is now an urgent need for the issue of genetic counselling to be considered. A few of the large research-based memory clinics already provide this service as part of their total work-up of the patient, as important as the history, examination and high technology scans. Genetic engineering has arrived for some diseases, could it have a role in the future in chronic confusion?

Despite the major advances in medicine and science, the reality for most people is of a slow decline into a mental desert, dependent on their loved ones for care and comfort. Carers above all need hope, but even more they deserve recognition of their role and as much practical support as they feel they need. It is a cliché that knowledge is power, but with dementia there are at least two victims, sufferer and carer, and I hope that this book helps both.

Conclusion

The number of very old people in our society is set to increase rapidly into the next century. All carers will then face enormous difficulties that will only be overcome with a close degree of partnership. The increasing number of people living to old age is, and must be seen to be by society, a success story. The fact that the elderly are more prone to lots of different illnesses should not detract from this. Most elderly people live completely fit and independent lives. For those that do fall ill much can be done, and for most the condition can be cured or substantially alleviated.

Chronic conditions by their very nature will always be with the elderly in one form or another. To accept this fact as inevitably leading to dependence is wrong. Active rehabilitation can postpone dependence indefinitely, remembering that dependence in old age is not due to old age but to ill health. The aim must be to envisage old age as a time of enjoyment, with health problems tackled as vigorously as in the young. There will always be some for whom early and accurate diagnosis, full treatment and rehabilitation will be insufficient and in whom the underlying disease process will continue. This is certainly true of Alzheimer's dementia. However there is some evidence that a caring environment accompanied by techniques such as reality orientation can postpone further rapid deterioration so that the disease only progresses gradually, leaving most sufferers a good quality of life for many years.

It is to be hoped that, with continuing public and professional education, 'ageism' in all areas diminishes. It is morally wrong and financially absurd to spend vast sums of money on a large group of people at the end of their disease process, placing them in institutions instead of ensuring prevention and early detection of disease. The old have as valid and worthy a stake in preventive medicine as any other age group. The pendulum has a long way to swing before the elderly receive the same kind of publicity associated with, say, child immunisation projects, child abuse, AIDS, smoking, etc. All are important. Why are the elderly less important than others?

Parts of this awareness and consciousness-raising of health issues in the elderly will inevitably lead to more preventive work and early recognition of diseases by the primary health care team – GPs, nurses, health visitors, etc. This means that all health care professionals will have to keep abreast of current developments in all fields of health care in the elderly. The GP is a vital and powerful gatekeeper when it comes to the early detection and treatment of ill health in old age; this is especially the case in confusional states, where delay in diagnosis can be disastrous.

Education concerning health matters is needed not only at all professional levels but also in the lay press. If glossy magazines were to publish as many articles on the early recognition of conditions that may cause confusional states or other medical conditions common in the elderly as they do articles on how to detect breast lumps, they may well increase their circulation. They would also provide insight and knowledge to at least three generations of women instead of the one or two generations they aim at now – the children and grandchildren of our current elderly.

For many the present and future dilemma is how to cope with a relative with dementia. To cope adequately a carer must under-stand the condition and how it may progress. It means knowing what to do in certain circumstances and where to go for practical help, advice and support. It means having a network of both professional and informal help, of not coping with the burden alone. Coping means knowing the law, getting the entitlements and most importantly it means understanding the system to get the information, the help and the support.

The caring continues as it always has done – there appears to be no decline in these acts of self-sacrifice. And it will continue as long as the carers are met at least halfway by the state. The provision of fundamental information and practical help with the caring role, and support during emotional strain, family upheavals, etc., can come from both statutory and voluntary concerns. The statutory sector, however, cannot shirk its responsibilities and expect the voluntary sector to pick up all the pieces. The role of the carer and all its implications have to be publicly recognised by the state and due credit given. Financial help must be widened and increased, because the caring performed by individuals is not only beyond price; it is beyond the capabilities of any health service to match, no matter how that service is funded.

For too long the care of the elderly in all aspects has been known as a Cinderella specialty. It is time for Cinders to go to the ball and for the clock to remain perpetually at one minute to midnight. Fairy godmothers may be a bit hard to come by, but dedication, commitment and a pride in the work is available in abundance.

The medical and social difficulties associated with old age will not go away; indeed they will increase. We know the problems and we have the solutions. All that is needed is the social and political commitment and then perhaps most of us will have a happier old age.

Further reading

Alzheimer's Disease Alzheimer's Disease Society, London

Caring for Elderly People – Understanding and Practical Help
Susan Hooker, Routledge & Kegan Paul, London

Caring for an Elderly Relative
Dr Keith Thompson, Vermilion, London

Caring for the Person with Dementia
Alzheimer's Disease Society

Coping at Home
Nancy Kohner, King's Fund Centre & National Extension College,
London & Cambridge

Dementia and Mental Illness in the Old
Elaine Murphy, Macmillan, London

The Law and Vulnerable Elderly People
edited by Sally Greengross, Age Concern, London

Nursing the Aged
Pat Young, Woodhead Faulkner, Cambridge

Taking Care of Your Elderly Relative
Dr J.A. Muir Gray and Heather Mackenzie, Penguin, London

The 36-Hour Day: Caring at Home for Confused Elderly People
Mace, Rabins, Cloke and McEwen, Age Concern, London

Who Cares?
Health Education Authority, London

Useful Addresses

Age Concern Greater London
54 Knatchbull Road
London SE5 9QU
0171 274 6723

Age Concern Wales
1 Cathedral Road
Cardiff CF1 9SD
01222 371566

Age Concern Scotland
54A Fountain Bridge
Edinburgh EH3 9PT
0131 228 5656

Age Concern Northern Ireland
3 Lower Crescent
Belfast BT7 1NR
01232 245729

Alzheimer's Disease Society
2nd Floor, Gordon House
10 Greencoat Place
London SW1P 1PH
0171 306 0606

Association of Continence Advisers
Disabled Living Foundation
380-4 Harrow Road
London W9 2HU
0171 266 3704

British Association of Occupational Therapists
6 Marshalsea Road
London SE1 1HL
0171 357 6480

British Geriatrics Society (BGS)
1 St Andrews Place
Regents Park
London NW1 4LB
0171 935 4004

British Red Cross
9 Grosvenor Crescent
London SW1X 7EJ
0171 235 5454

Campaign for Single Homeless People (CHAR)
5-15 Cromer Street
London WC1
0171 833 2071

Centre for Policy on Ageing (CPA)
25-31 Ironmonger Row
London EC1V 3QP
0171 253 1787

Chartered Society of Physiotherapy
14 Bedford Row
London WC1R 4ED
0171 242 1941

Community Service Volunteers
237 Pentonville Road
Kings Cross
London N1 9NG
0171 278 6001

Counsel and Care for the Elderly
Twyman House
24 Kingsway
London WC2B 6HD
0171 485 1550

Court of Protection
Stewart House
24 Kingsway
London WC2B 6HD
0171 269 7000

Disability Alliance
Universal House
Wentworth Street
London E1 7SA
0171 289 8776

Disabled Living Foundation
380-4 Harrow Road
London W9 2HU
0171 289 6111

Health Education Authority
Hamilton House
Mabledon Place
London WC1
0171 387 9528

Help the Aged
St James' Walk
London EC1R 0BE
0171 253 0253

Jewish Care
221 Golders Green Road
London NW11 9DZ
0181 458 3282

King's Fund Centre
126 Albert Street
London NW1 7NF
0171 267 6111

MIND - National Association for
Mental Health
22 Harley Street
London W1N 2ED
0171 637 0741

National Association of Citizens
Advice Bureaux
115 Pentonville Road
London N1 9LZ
0171 833 2181

National Council for Voluntary
Organisations (NCVO)
26 Bedford Square
London WC1B 3HU
0171 636 4066

Parkinson's Disease Society
36 Portland Street
London W1N 3DG
0171 383 3513

Royal Association for Disability
and Rehabilitation (RADAR)
25 Mortimer Street
London W1N 8AB
0171 637 5400

Royal National Institute for the Blind
224 Great Portland Street
London W1N 4XX
0171 388 1266

Shape
1 Thorpe Close
London W10 5XL
0181 960 9245

St Johns Ambulance
1 Grosvenor Crescent
London SW1X 7EE
0171 235 5231

Talking Books for the Handicapped (National Listening Library)
12 Lant Street
London SE1 1QH
0171 407 9417

Terrence Higgins Trust
52/54 Gray's Inn Road
London WC1X 8JU
0171 242 1010 (12 noon - 7 pm every day)

Index

Page numbers in *italics* refer to illustrations.

questionnaires, 45–6, 110–11

Registered Home Act, 124
research, 133–40
residential homes, 83–5, 93–5
risks, 53–4
Royal London Hospital (Mile End), 105, 109–110

Section 47, 115
sedatives, 12–13
senile dementia of the Alzheimer type, (SDAT), 43
sexual behaviour, 52–3
sight, 22–3
sitting services, 85–6
skin infections, 17–19, *18*
sleep, 51–2
social embarrassment, 49–50
social policy, 3–4
social workers, 81–2, 84, 90, 130, 131
speech difficulties, 50–1
staffing levels, old people's homes, 84
stairs, 88

state benefits, 89–92
steroids, 13
strokes, 15–16, 65–9
swallowing, 67–8
syphilis, 30–1

telephone alarm system, 86
Terrence Higgins Trust, 119
thyroid gland, 27–9
tranquillisers, 12–13

ulcers, 17–18, *18*
University College Hospital, London, 105, 107
urinary tract infection, 8–10, 23

viruses, 138–9
vitamin B12 deficiency, 29–30
voluntary and community groups, 92–3
voluntary help organisations, 72
vomiting, 17

will, living, 118–20